AF838006

Individualized Treatment Strategies in the Radiotherapy Era

Over the years, radiation therapy has had both remarkable successes in saving lives and a number of silent struggles for the patient. This text is not about turning away from radiation therapy; it's about using it thoughtfully and recognizing that not every patient needs the same path. In an era where oncology is moving rapidly towards personalization, radiation therapy should have evidence-driven use. The editors and authors have brought together evolving ideas, research and case experiences to help clinicians think differently, treating each patient as an individual, not just as a diagnosis, and to invite them to pause, to question and to reimagine how to plan treatment—always with the patient's best interests at heart. This book will serve as a guide for oncologists, radiation specialists, surgeons and clinical researchers, providing new frameworks for integrating no radiation therapy (NO-RT) strategies into modern cancer care.

Individualized Treatment Strategies in the Radiotherapy Era

No-RT and Beyond RT

Edited by
Shrikant Khare, MD
Department of Radiotherapy
Regional Referral Hospital
Nashik, India

Rahul Jain, MS, MBA, PGD QA
Department of Gastroenterology
Hematology & Oncology
VSG Group of Companies
Nashik, India

Vishal Gulecha, PhD
Shree Panchvati Education Society's
Smt Narmadaben Popatlal Thakkar Institute of Pharmacy
Nashik, India

Rahul Sapate, BSc, PGD CN
Department of Gastroenterology
Hematology & Oncology
VSG Group of Companies
Nashik, India

CRC Press
Taylor & Francis Group
Boca Raton London New York

CRC Press is an imprint of the
Taylor & Francis Group, an **informa** business

Designed cover image: Shutterstock

First edition published 2026
by CRC Press
2385 NW Executive Center Drive, Suite 320, Boca Raton, FL 33431

and by CRC Press
4 Park Square, Milton Park, Abingdon, Oxon, OX14 4RN

CRC Press is an imprint of Taylor & Francis Group, LLC

© 2026 selection and editorial matter, Shrikant Khare, Rahul Jain, Rahul Sapate and Vishal Gulecha
individual chapters, the contributors

This book contains information obtained from authentic and highly regarded sources. While all reasonable efforts have been made to publish reliable data and information, neither the author[s] nor the publisher can accept any legal responsibility or liability for any errors or omissions that may be made. The publishers wish to make clear that any views or opinions expressed in this book by individual editors, authors or contributors are personal to them and do not necessarily reflect the views/opinions of the publishers. The information or guidance contained in this book is intended for use by medical, scientific or health-care professionals and is provided strictly as a supplement to the medical or other professional's own judgement, their knowledge of the patient's medical history, relevant manufacturer's instructions and the appropriate best practice guidelines. Because of the rapid advances in medical science, any information or advice on dosages, procedures or diagnoses should be independently verified. The reader is strongly urged to consult the relevant national drug formulary and the drug companies' and device or material manufacturers' printed instructions, and their websites, before administering or utilizing any of the drugs, devices or materials mentioned in this book. This book does not indicate whether a particular treatment is appropriate or suitable for a particular individual. Ultimately it is the sole responsibility of the medical professional to make his or her own professional judgements, so as to advise and treat patients appropriately. The authors and publishers have also attempted to trace the copyright holders of all material reproduced in this publication and apologize to copyright holders if permission to publish in this form has not been obtained. If any copyright material has not been acknowledged please write and let us know so we may rectify in any future reprint.

Except as permitted under U.S. Copyright Law, no part of this book may be reprinted, reproduced, transmitted, or utilized in any form by any electronic, mechanical, or other means, now known or hereafter invented, including photocopying, microfilming, and recording, or in any information storage or retrieval system, without written permission from the publishers.

For permission to photocopy or use material electronically from this work, access www.copyright.com or contact the Copyright Clearance Center, Inc. (CCC), 222 Rosewood Drive, Danvers, MA 01923, 978-750-8400. For works that are not available on CCC please contact mpkbookspermissions@tandf.co.uk

For Product Safety Concerns and Information please contact our EU representative GPSR@taylorandfrancis.com. Taylor & Francis Verlag GmbH, Kaufingerstraße 24, 80331 München, Germany.

Trademark notice: Product or corporate names may be trademarks or registered trademarks and are used only for identification and explanation without intent to infringe.

ISBN: 9781032867656 (hbk)
ISBN: 9781032867649 (pbk)
ISBN: 9781003529071 (ebk)

DOI: 10.1201/9781003529071

Typeset in Minion
by KnowledgeWorks Global Ltd.

Contents

Preface, vii

Acknowledgements, ix

Contributors, xi

Chapter 1 ▪ Introducing the NO-RT Concept and Changing Treatment Paradigms 1

Shrikant Khare, Rahul Jain, Rahul Sapate and Vishal Gulecha

Chapter 2 ▪ Recognizing Tumour Biology and Assessing Radiation Therapy Need 20

Mangesh Korde and Mukesh Chandra

Chapter 3 ▪ Surgical Aspects: Examining Surgery's Significance in Tumour Management 49

Nagesh Madnoorkar and Shantanu Pawar

Chapter 4 ▪ Alternative Modalities: Assessing Treatment Choices Other Than Radiation 62

Peeyush Shukla, Rahul Sapate and Sandeep Ishi

Chapter 5 ▪ Patient Selection Standards: Recognizing Potential NO-RT Candidates 76

Peeyush Shukla and Shrikant Khare

Chapter 6 ▪ Clinical Determination: Handling Therapy Algorithms 89

Pooja Thakare and Gagandipsingh Bhamra

Chapter 7 ▪ Case Studies: Showing Effective Uses of NO-RT Principles 111

Shrikant Khare, Peeyush Shukla and Shantanu Pawar

Chapter 8 ▪ Difficulties and Disputations: Handling Issues and Discussions in the Domain 123

Rahul Jain, Rahul Sapate and Vishal Gulecha

Chapter 9 ▪ Multidisciplinary Cooperation: Combining Viewpoints to Provide the Best Possible Patient Care 136

Lalesh Nahata, Vaishali Khare, Nagesh Madnoorkar, Shrikant Khare and Rahul Jain

Chapter 10 ▪ Concluding Remarks: Using NO-RT in a Holistic Cancer Treatment Approach 151

Rahul Jain, Rahul Sapate and Vishal Gulecha

INDEX, 159

Preface

OVER THE YEARS, WORKING AS A RADIATION ONCOLOGIST, I have witnessed both the remarkable successes and the silent struggles that come with radiation therapy. There is no denying that it has saved countless lives. But as oncology advances, I found myself wondering: Are there times when less could actually be more for our patients? Through many conversations with colleagues and reflections drawn from clinical experience, the idea for this book, *Individualized Treatment Strategies in the Radiotherapy Era: No-RT and Beyond RT*, began to take shape. It isn't about turning away from radiation therapy; it's about using it thoughtfully and recognizing that not every patient needs the same path.

This book was born from a simple but profound question: In an era where oncology is moving rapidly towards personalization, why does radiation therapy often remain a default? This book is not a rejection of radiation therapy but a call for its optimized, evidence-driven use. In these pages, we have tried to bring together evolving ideas, research and case experiences to help doctors think differently—to treat each patient as an individual, not just as a diagnosis.

Our hope is that this book invites you to pause, to question and to reimagine how we plan treatment—always with the patient's best interests at heart. We hope it serves as a guide for oncologists, radiation specialists, surgeons and clinical researchers, providing new frameworks for integrating NO-RT strategies into modern cancer care.

Shrikant Khare

Acknowledgements

THERE ARE SO MANY PEOPLE without whom this work would never have reached these pages.

I would like to specially thank the team of contributors who walked alongside us in this journey: Dr Nagesh Madnoorkar, Dr Mangesh Korde, Dr Mukesh Chandre, Dr Piyush Shukla, Dr Shantanu Pawar, Dr Lalesh Nahata, Dr Sandeep Ishi, Dr Vaishali Khare, Pooja Thakare and Gagandipsingh Bhamra. Their experience, hard-earned knowledge and, above all, willingness to share and collaborate made a real difference. This book has many voices behind it, and each one of them helped shape it into something better than we could have managed alone; we thank Regional Referral Service Hospital, Nashik; Chopda Medicare & Research Centre Pvt. Ltd.; Magnum Heart Institute Nashik; and VSG Group of Companies for standing behind us with their encouragement and trust.

I would also like to acknowledge Dr Manoj Chopda and Dr Vaibhav Gulecha, whose guidance and steady support were a great source of strength during the preparation of this book.

And finally, to our patients—every story, every journey and every challenge they face remind us why we must keep questioning, keep learning and keep striving for better care.

Shrikant Khare

Contributors

Gagandipsingh Bhamra
Department of Oncology
Newcastle University
Newcastle upon Tyne, United Kingdom

Mukesh Chandra
Department of Radiotherapy
Kalyan Cancer Centre
Kalyan, India

Sandeep Ishi
NIMS Hospital
Nashik, India

Vaishali Khare
Maya Superspeciality Clinic
Nashik, India

Mangesh Korde
Department of Radiotherapy
Nashik Cancer Centre
Nashik, India

Nagesh Madnoorkar
Department of Surgical Oncology
Chopda Medicare & Research Centre Pvt. Ltd.
Magnum Heart Institute
Nashik, India

Lalesh Nahata
Department of Radiology
Matrix Scan Centre
Nashik, India

Shantanu Pawar
Department of Surgical Oncology
Regional Referral Hospital
Nashik, India

Peeyush Shukla
Department of Radiotherapy
International Oncology Cancer Institute (IOCI)
Indore, India

Pooja Thakare
Department of Gastroenterology, Hematology & Oncology
VSG Group of Companies
Nashik, India

CHAPTER 1

Introducing the NO-RT Concept and Changing Treatment Paradigms

Shrikant Khare, Rahul Jain, Rahul Sapate and Vishal Gulecha

OVERVIEW OF RADIATION THERAPY

Radiation therapy (RT) has been a cornerstone of cancer treatment for over a century. More than 14 million new cases of cancer are diagnosed annually worldwide. RT plays an important role in the management of these cancers. According to conservative estimates, RT can improve the cure rates of 3.5 million people and provide palliative relief to an additional 3.5 million (Barton et al., 2006; Tyldesley et al., 2011; Barton et al., 2014; Jaffray & Gospodarowicz, 2015). Approximately half of all cancer patients can benefit from RT, with about half of these presenting early enough for curative treatment. The use of RT in cancer treatment began with the discovery of X-rays by Wilhelm Conrad Roentgen in 1895. X-rays were applied for the first time in cancer treatment after this discovery, especially when E.H. Grubb treated a breast cancer patient (Lederman, 1981; Huh & Kim, 2020). This was considered the birth of RT. In the early days, T. Stenbeck and T. Sjögren began using X-rays to treat skin cancers. By 1903, RT was also used to treat leukaemia (Holsti, 1995). Doctors in France started using RT to treat stomach cancer in 1896 and achieved some pain relief and disease improvement (Huh & Kim, 2020). In 1902 Guido Holzknecht of Austria developed the first Roentgen-based dosimetry system. Using a chromoradiometer, the radiation doses were measured by observing colour changes in a salt mixture, a precursor to modern dosimetry systems (Thames, 1988). Dosimetry determines the correct radiation dose and is now an important aspect of radiation treatment. By the mid-20th century, proper dosimetry systems were developed, and the introduction of cobalt-60 (Co-60) beam therapy in the 1950s and 1960s marked the first significant improvement in RT technology (Buschke, 1970). Today, RT is a fundamental part of cancer care globally regardless of the economic status of a country. It is used in various applications, including curative treatment for localized cancers and palliative care for advanced or disseminated cancers (Jaffray & Gospodarowicz, 2015). RT is often combined with surgery either pre- or postoperatively

DOI: 10.1201/9781003529071-1

and also in systemic chemotherapy to improve its effectiveness (Barton et al., 2014). The main principle behind RT is controlled doses of ionizing radiation to damage the DNA of cancer cells. This process commonly affects cancer cells more compared to normal tissues, which makes it effective in treating a wide range of cancer types. However, ensuring the therapeutic ratio that balances tumour control and avoiding unacceptable toxicity in normal tissues require precise control over radiation doses. Less than a 5% deviation in dose delivery can be tolerated. However, there is a need for specialized equipment and a highly trained team, including radiation oncologists, medical physicists and technologists (Gospodarowicz et al., 2015). RT can cure localized cancers, control advanced ones and provide palliative care in oncology.

INTRODUCTION TO NO-RT

The concept of no radiation therapy (NO-RT) in oncology has emerged as a significant approach. This approach mainly aims to improve patient outcomes by minimizing the use of radiation in cancer treatment. This method was made possible due to the advances in surgical techniques, targeted therapies and systemic treatments that provide effective cancer control without the need for radiation. NO-RT is relevant in cases where radiation may cause unnecessary risks or compromise the quality of life (QoL). Hence this NO-RT method provides an alternative that emphasizes long-term health and patient-centred care.

Recent discoveries in cancer surgery and treatment modalities have made NO-RT a useful option in certain cancer treatment methods. For example, advances in minimally invasive surgical techniques have successfully removed tumours with fewer side effects and less reliance on radiation in certain cancers (Datta et al., 2024). Moreover, the advances in targeted therapies where the cancer cells are attacked specifically based on their genetic or molecular profiles have shown efficacy in treating cancers that may need RT. This often reduces the treatment burden and associated adverse effects (Turner, 2024). A focus of NO-RT is the improvement in the patient's QoL. This approach is supported by studies indicating that patients who choose non-invasive treatments, including NO-RT, often reported improved health-related QoL (Wolf, 2023). Additionally, research demonstrates that forgoing radiation can result in comparable long-term survival outcomes while reducing complications such as radiation-induced toxicity and secondary malignancies. However, it is important to understand that NO-RT is not suitable for all cancer types. So a careful evaluation of individual patient circumstances is essential to ensure the most effective treatment plan is selected. Patient selection is crucial when determining the necessity of RT. The LUMINA-(omitting radiotherapy after breast-conserving surgery in luminal a breast cancer) trial demonstrated that older patients (≥55 years) with low-risk luminal A breast cancer defined by small, hormone receptor-positive, HER2-negative tumours may safely omit RT following breast-conserving surgery and endocrine therapy. With a 5-year local recurrence rate of only 2.3%, this subgroup can avoid the potential side effects of RT without compromising outcomes (Whelan et al., 2023). Conversely, younger patients with triple-negative breast cancer (TNBC) typically require RT due to the aggressive nature of TNBC and its higher recurrence risk. Studies have shown that adjuvant RT significantly improves survival and reduces recurrence rates, particularly when combined with chemotherapy. Similarly, in rectal cancer, findings from the OPRA (organ preservation in patients with rectal adenocarcinoma) trial support a selective approach, where patients achieving a clinical complete response after total neoadjuvant therapy (TNT) may forgo surgery and RT, while those with residual disease still require intervention. These examples highlight the shift towards individualized treatment strategies, ensuring that patients receive RT only when its benefits outweigh the risks. Personalized approaches based on tumour biology, patient demographics and treatment response are essential for optimizing outcomes while minimizing unnecessary exposure to RT (De Santis et al., 2024).

The NO-RT approach is an evolving paradigm in oncology that seeks to optimize patient outcomes by reducing or eliminating the need for RT when feasible. This strategy is supported by advances in surgical techniques, targeted therapies and systemic treatments, which can effectively control cancer while minimizing the risks associated with radiation.

The shift away from RT has also been facilitated by advancements in minimally invasive surgical techniques, which allow for precise tumour removal with minimal damage to surrounding tissues (Datta et al., 2024). In addition, targeted therapies that exploit genetic and molecular markers, such as HER2-targeted agents and immune checkpoint inhibitors, have demonstrated effectiveness in reducing tumour burden and recurrence risks, thereby decreasing reliance on radiation (Turner, 2024). Research has shown that patients undergoing NO-RT experience improved health-related QoL, avoiding complications like radiation-induced toxicity, fatigue and secondary malignancies (Wolf, 2023). However, NO-RT is not universally applicable, and a careful, evidence-based approach is essential to determine the most appropriate treatment plan for each patient (De Santis et al., 2024).

CHANGING PARADIGMS

The evolving landscape of oncology can be observed by a significant shift towards NO-RT. This is driven by advancements in diagnostics, surgical techniques, systemic therapies and a growing focus on patient-centred care. This paradigm shift is reshaping traditional cancer treatment approaches by emphasizing personalized, targeted therapies that aim to reduce the burden of radiation on patients while maintaining or improving treatment outcomes as illustrated in **Figure 1.1**.

The development of advanced imaging technologies and molecular profiling has significantly improved early cancer detection. This allows clinicians to design more tailored treatment plans that may exclude RT. Novel in vitro diagnostics and in vivo imaging also improve the ability to monitor disease progression and further reduce the necessity of radiation in some cases (De Jong et al., 2023; Liu et al., 2023). These innovations contribute to more effective treatment decisions and help in the rise of NO-RT. Minimally invasive surgical techniques have advanced significantly, allowing for more precise tumour resections with fewer complications. These surgical improvements have decreased the need for adjunctive RT. This is because complete resections often reduce the risk of cancer recurrence (Turgeman & Ben-Aharon, 2021).

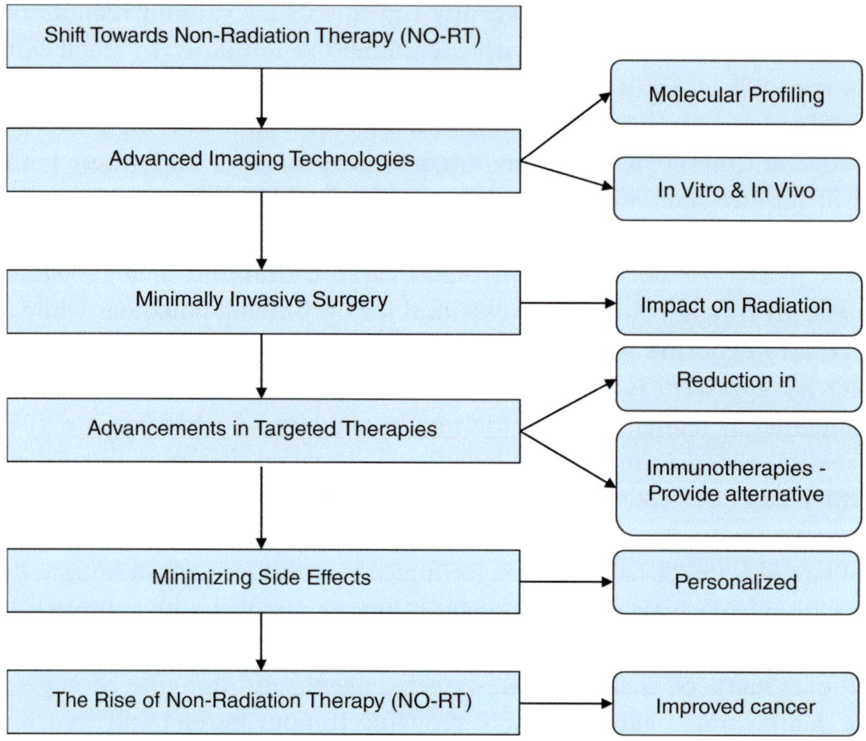

FIGURE 1.1 Changing paradigm to NO-RT.

Surgical outcomes improve the feasibility of NO-RT as an option in comprehensive cancer care (Premnath & Madanat, 2023). The advancements in targeted therapies and immunotherapies have transformed cancer treatment methods by providing alternatives to radiation in many cases. Targeted agents that specifically address genetic mutations in cancers such as non-small cell lung cancer have shown encouraging results. This enables more patients to avoid RT (De Jong et al., 2023; Liu et al., 2023). A growing interest in minimizing treatment side effects and improving post-treatment QoL has been a driving force behind the shift towards NO-RT. Personalized treatment plans that are supported by patient advocacy are increasingly prioritizing approaches that balance effectiveness with minimizing long-term radiation exposure (Turgeman & Ben-Aharon, 2021; Premnath & Madanat, 2023). The journey of evolution of radiotherapy and the rise of the No-RT approach, along with its advancements in disease management, improved patient quality of life, and avoidance of adverse events caused by unnecessary exposure to radiation therapy, is illustrated in **Figure 1.2**.

The development of advanced imaging technologies and molecular profiling has significantly improved early cancer detection. This allows clinicians to design more tailored treatment plans that may exclude radiation therapy. Novel in vitro diagnostics and in vivo imaging also improve the ability to monitor disease progression and further reduce the necessity of radiation in some cases (De Jong et al., 2023; Liu et al., 2023).

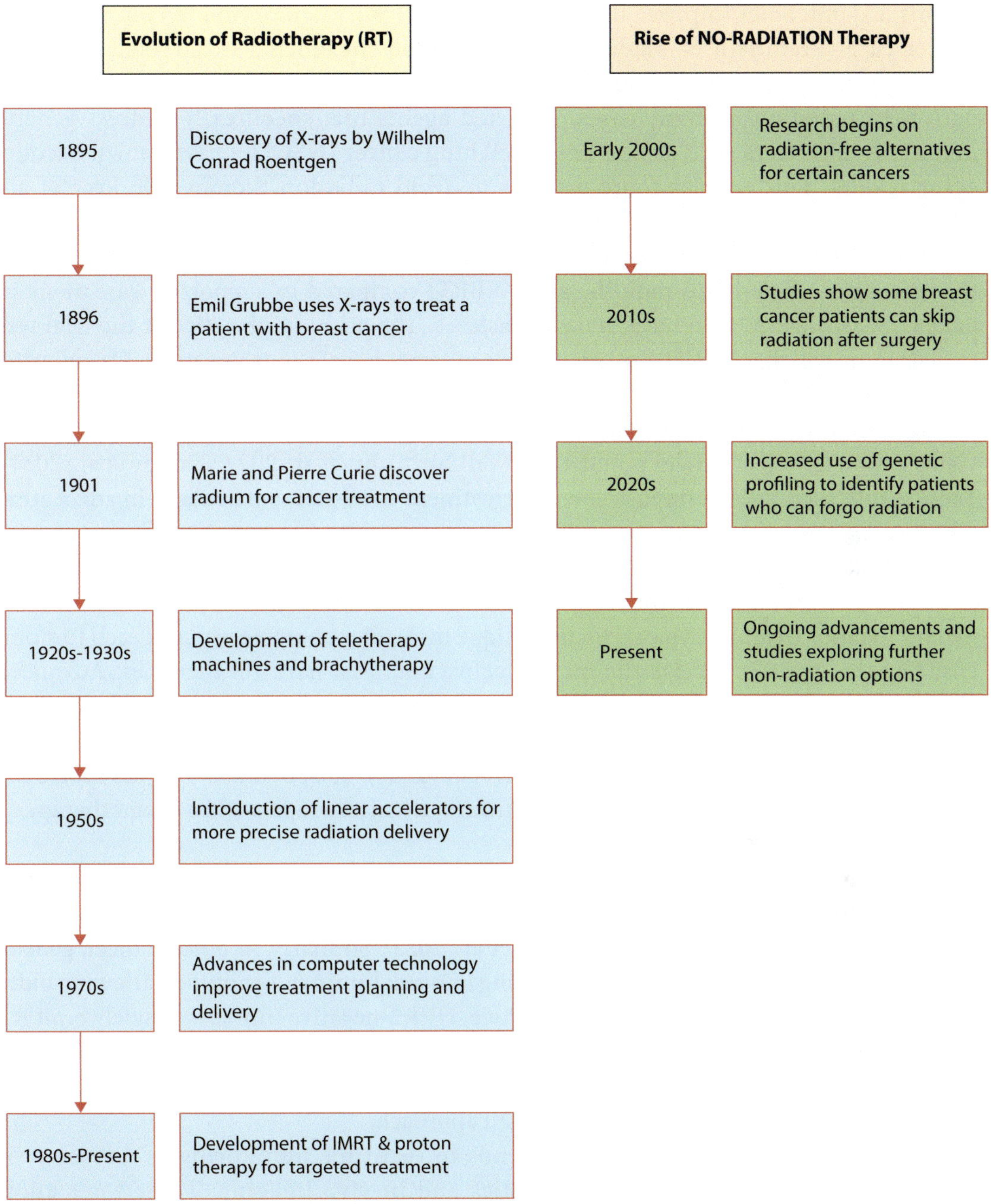

FIGURE 1.2 Evolution of radiotherapy and NO-RT.

These innovations contribute to more effective treatment decisions and help in the rise of NO-RT. Minimally invasive surgical techniques have advanced significantly, allowing for more precise tumour resections with fewer complications. These surgical improvements have decreased the need for adjunctive radiation therapy. This is because complete resections often reduce the risk of cancer recurrence (Turgeman & Ben-Aharon, 2021).

As surgical outcomes improve the feasibility of NO-RT as an option in comprehensive cancer care (Premnath & Madanat, 2023). The advancements in targeted therapies and immunotherapies have transformed cancer treatment methods by providing alternatives to radiation in many cases. Targeted agents that specifically address genetic mutations in cancers such as non-small cell lung cancer (NSCLC) have shown encouraging results. This enables more patients to avoid radiation therapy (De Jong et al., 2023; Liu et al., 2023).

The QUARTZ trial was a pivotal phase 3, non-inferiority study designed to assess the efficacy of whole-brain radiotherapy (WBRT) compared to supportive care alone in patients with NSCLC who have brain metastases. The primary objective of the trial was to determine whether WBRT provided any significant benefit in terms of quality-adjusted life years (QALYs), overall survival (OS) or QoL. The findings indicated that WBRT did not significantly improve these outcomes, suggesting that supportive care alone could be a viable option for select patient populations (Trikhirhisthit et al., 2022; Starkey et al., 2024). These results have crucial implications for treatment strategies, particularly in advocating for a NO-RT approach in specific cases.

Personalized treatment plans are revolutionizing cancer care, especially as NO-RT strategies gain prominence. The integration of biomarkers and genetic profiling allows clinicians to tailor treatments based on the unique molecular characteristics of each tumour, ensuring that patients receive the most effective and least harmful therapies. Advanced molecular profiling can identify specific genetic mutations, receptor status and signalling pathways that not only influence tumour behaviour but also predict responsiveness to various treatments (De Jong et al., 2023; Liu et al., 2023). Such detailed insights enable the selection of patients who may benefit more from systemic therapies—like chemotherapy or targeted agents—instead of traditional RT.

For instance, in NSCLC, patients with mutations in genes such as *EGFR* or *ALK* have shown favourable responses to targeted therapies, resulting in improved survival outcomes and reduced toxicity compared to RT (Liu et al., 2023). Similarly, in breast cancer, genetic profiling has been instrumental in identifying low-risk luminal A subtypes, allowing older patients with small, hormone receptor-positive, HER2-negative tumours to safely omit RT after breast-conserving surgery and endocrine therapy (Whelan et al., 2023). These examples underscore the importance of individualized treatment, where decisions are guided by tumour biology rather than a one-size-fits-all approach.

Moreover, the role of biomarkers extends to real-time monitoring of disease progression through novel in vitro diagnostics and in vivo imaging. These tools allow for the dynamic adjustment of treatment plans based on changes in tumour genetics and patient response, further optimizing outcomes (Turgeman & Ben-Aharon, 2021). This patient-centred, biomarker-driven strategy not only enhances therapeutic efficacy but also improves QoL by minimizing exposure to the adverse effects of radiation. Ultimately, as emerging data continue to refine our understanding, personalized treatment plans will play a critical role in determining the appropriateness of NO-RT approaches, guiding precision oncology towards safer and more effective care (Premnath & Madanat, 2023).

TRIAL DESIGN AND KEY OUTCOMES

The QUARTZ trial was structured as a non-inferiority trial, comparing the outcomes of patients receiving WBRT plus supportive care to those receiving supportive care alone. The primary endpoints included QALYs, OS, and QoL measures. The study enrolled patients with NSCLC and brain metastases who were not candidates for surgery or stereotactic radiosurgery (SRS) due to disease burden or performance status (Starkey et al., 2024).

The results demonstrated no significant improvement in QALYs or OS for patients receiving WBRT compared to those who did not. Median OS was similar between the two groups, indicating that WBRT did not provide a meaningful survival advantage (Trikhirhisthit et al., 2022). Additionally, patients in the WBRT group experienced higher toxicity and neurocognitive decline without corresponding improvements in symptom control or QoL (Nieder et al., 2020). These findings prompted a re-evaluation of WBRT's necessity in certain NSCLC patients with brain metastases, particularly those with poor prognostic factors.

SUPPORT FOR NO-RT STRATEGY

The QUARTZ trial provides strong evidence supporting a NO-RT strategy in select patient populations, particularly those with poor performance status or limited life expectancy, where the potential benefits of WBRT do not outweigh the associated risks and side effects (Starkey et al., 2024). This approach aligns with the broader movement towards de-escalation of radiotherapy in cases where treatment-related morbidity outweighs potential benefits (Trikhirhisthit et al., 2022). Additionally, the decision to omit WBRT can be particularly relevant for patients with significant extracranial disease or those not eligible for aggressive treatments. The trial's findings reinforce the necessity of individualized treatment plans, incorporating factors such as patient prognosis, symptoms and the availability of systemic therapies that might control brain metastases more effectively (Nieder et al., 2020).

COMPLEMENTARY TRIALS AND EMERGING DATA

The trend towards de-escalation of radiotherapy is further supported by complementary trials. The ENCEPHALON trial, which compared stereotactic radiotherapy (SRT) to WBRT in small cell lung cancer (SCLC) patients, found that SRT was associated with better neurocognitive outcomes without compromising survival (Bernhardt et al., 2023). These findings emphasize the growing preference for targeted radiotherapy approaches over WBRT in specific patient groups.

Furthermore, emerging data from immuno-oncology studies suggest that systemic therapies such as immune checkpoint inhibitors may offer survival benefits comparable to or exceeding those of WBRT. Studies indicate that immunotherapy and targeted therapies could allow for the omission of WBRT in certain patients while maintaining disease control (Starkey et al., 2024). Additionally, precision oncology approaches have identified molecular subtypes of NSCLC with brain metastases that may respond better to systemic therapies than radiotherapy alone (Wong et al., 2024).

While the QUARTZ trial and related studies provide compelling evidence for considering a NO-RT strategy in NSCLC patients with brain metastases, treatment decisions must remain individualized. Factors such as patient performance status, genetic mutations and the presence of extracranial disease should guide therapy selection. Moreover, the availability of effective systemic therapies further supports the omission of WBRT in select cases. However, continued evaluation of WBRT's role across diverse patient populations remains essential, considering cultural and regional variations in treatment outcomes (Ng et al., 2019).

CASE FOR NO-RT

The use of NO-RT in select cases of pancreatic cancer has shown promising results in improving patient outcomes. Some studies have stated that even if radiotherapy can help in controlling the local tumour, it also has risks like toxicity and adverse effects that may outweigh the benefits in certain populations. Improved systemic chemotherapy and targeted therapies can also help in controlling the progression of disease and improving the QoL. For example Cao et al. (2023) and other similar studies observed that advanced chemotherapy alone without using radiotherapy has allowed for the management of tumours and increased the survival in inoperable pancreatic cancer cases significantly. These approaches have reduced treatment-related complications like gastrointestinal toxicity and damage to surrounding organs that are commonly associated with radiotherapy. Systemic therapy without RT is related to better management of distant metastases. It is an essential consideration, given the high rates of distant progression in pancreatic cancer. Additionally, patients with favourable prognostic markers like lower CA19-9 levels and early-stage diagnoses can benefit from NO-RT strategies, experiencing improved progression-free survival (PFS) and OS.

Over recent years the changing paradigm in the treatment of locally advanced rectal cancer (LARC) has emphasized minimizing the invasiveness of interventions to improve patient QoL. Avoiding radical surgical procedures in cases of complete clinical response (cCR) following neoadjuvant therapy (NAT) is increasingly supported by evidence. The advent of TNT has improved efficacy in treatment that results in high rates of cCR and pathological complete response (pCR). This advancement has led to the development of non-operative management (NOM) strategies, including the watch and wait (WW) protocol (Smith et al., 2015). Clinical data have shown that TNT has increased cCR rates significantly, and this enabled a considerable number of patients to choose NOM with active surveillance rather than undergoing total mesorectal excision (TME). Promising outcomes have been observed by avoiding TME, such as a decrease in the risks of post-surgical complications like problems in bowel, urinary and sexual functions. These problems were reported in over 80% of patients who undergo surgery. The OPRA trial has demonstrated that the preservation of organs is feasible in approximately 50% of patients treated with TNT. These findings have highlighted the significance of patient-centred approaches and informed decision-making. Thus, individualized treatment plans focus on oncological safety and QoL (Goffredo et al., 2022).

PRIME II Trial

The PRIME II trial investigated the necessity of postoperative RT in older women (≥65 years) with hormone receptor-positive, low-risk early breast cancer. The study found that while omitting RT led to a slight increase in local recurrence, it did not impact distant recurrence rates or OS. These findings suggest that for select patients, radiotherapy may be safely avoided without compromising long-term outcomes, thereby reducing treatment burden, side effects and healthcare costs (Kunkler et al., 2015). This evidence strengthens the rationale for a de-escalated treatment approach in low-risk breast cancer cases.

OPRA Trial

The OPRA trial provided crucial evidence for the feasibility of NOM in rectal cancer patients following TNT. The study demonstrated that patients achieving a cCR could safely forgo surgery, with outcomes comparable to those undergoing standard treatment. This approach resulted in reduced local recurrence rates and preserved organ function, significantly improving QoL. The trial supports the broader movement towards personalized, less invasive treatment strategies, reinforcing the concept that carefully selected patients can benefit from a NO-RT or NOM approach without compromising oncological outcomes (Thompson et al., 2024).

Some studies indicate that selected early-stage breast cancer patients, especially those over 70, have achieved survival rates with hormone therapy alone without any side effects that are associated with RT (Hughes et al., 2013). The PRIME II trial has stated that postoperative radiation in older patients with hormone receptor-positive, low-risk breast cancer did not significantly impact local recurrence rates or OS. This suggests that NO- RT can be a safe and effective approach in certain cases (Kunkler et al., 2015). Similarly, the research on prostate cancer management indicates that for men with low-risk disease, active surveillance and deferred radiation can help in the maintenance of QoL without any compromise in cancer-specific survival (Hamdy et al., 2016). Also, some comprehensive national data like New Zealand's Radiation Oncology Collection (ROC) highlight the need to personalize the treatment according to patients and the characteristics of the tumour to avoid unnecessary treatments (Imlach et al., 2023). All these examples state that NO-RT can be beneficial for patient outcomes when guided by proper patient selection and supported by data analysis. They can be fostered by personalized treatment plans that help in optimizing patient safety and resource usage.

STUDIES

Advanced chemotherapy has emerged as a pivotal strategy for managing tumours and improving survival in patients with advanced cancers while mitigating the risks of RT-related complications.

Study 1—FOLFIRINOX vs. Gemcitabine Alone

A systematic review and network meta-analysis comparing chemotherapy regimens for advanced pancreatic cancer found that FOLFIRINOX, a combination of 5-fluorouracil, leucovorin, irinotecan and oxaliplatin, significantly enhanced OS and PFS compared to gemcitabine alone (**Figure 1.3**). Despite its higher toxicity risk, FOLFIRINOX offered superior survival outcomes, underscoring the efficacy of aggressive chemotherapy in controlling tumour progression without requiring RT (Gresham et al., 2014).

Study 2—Gemcitabine Plus Nab-Paclitaxel

The combination of gemcitabine and nab-paclitaxel (Abraxane) has also demonstrated considerable advantages over gemcitabine alone in patients with advanced pancreatic cancer. Clinical trials revealed significant improvements in OS and PFS with this regimen, leading to its establishment as a standard first-line treatment. Importantly, these outcomes were achieved without the addition of RT, thereby avoiding potential RT-related complications (Gresham et al., 2014).

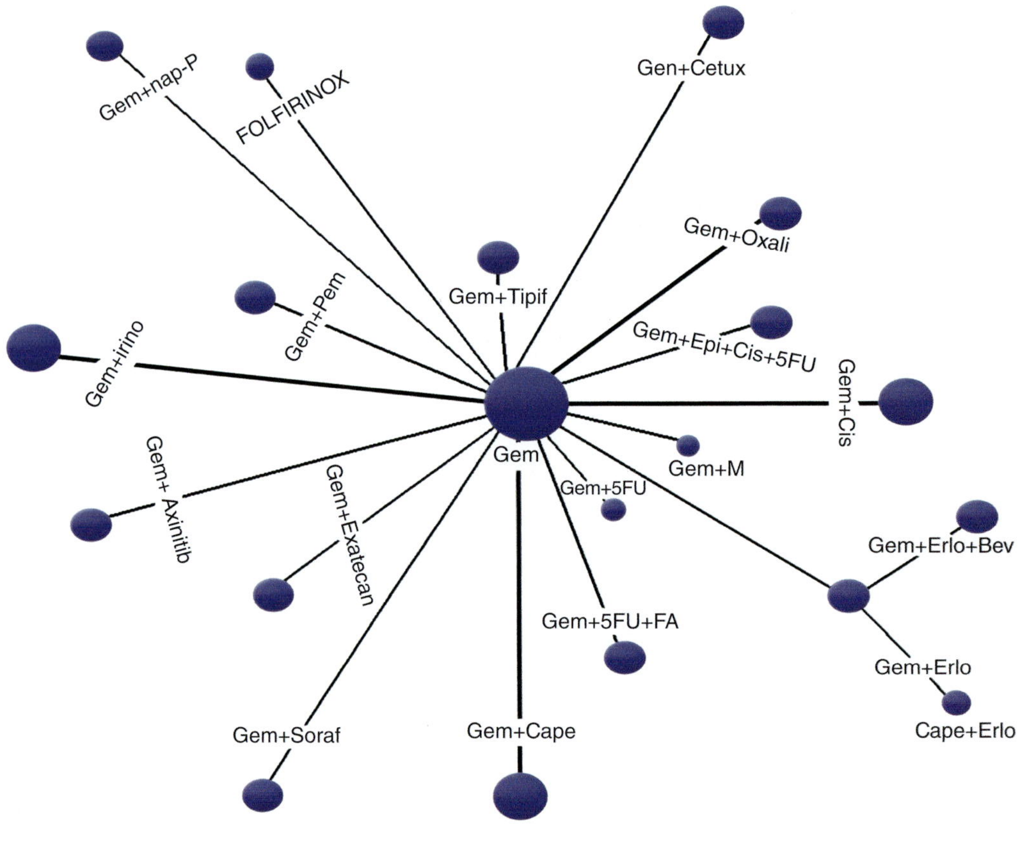

FIGURE 1.3 Illustrates the network of eligible trials comparing gemcitabine with other treatments. Circle size represents patient numbers, line thickness indicates trial count and distance from gemcitabine reflects publication year (1 cm = 2 years). (From Gresham et al. 2014 under Creative Commons Licence.)

Study 3—Real-World Study on Second-Line Chemotherapy

Studies on advanced chemotherapy demonstrate its capacity to manage tumours effectively and improve survival in advanced pancreatic adenocarcinoma (APC), reducing reliance on RT and avoiding associated complications. A pivotal real-world study comparing second-line chemotherapy to supportive care highlighted the potential of chemotherapy to extend survival without RT. Patients who received second-line chemotherapy had a median OS of 5.6 months compared to just 1.9 months for those on supportive care (hazard ratio [HR] = 0.766, 95% confidence interval [CI] = 0.677–0.867; $P < 0.001$). This underscores the significant survival advantage of chemotherapy in this population.

Further evidence supports the efficacy of specific regimens, such as gemcitabine- and 5-fluorouracil (5-FU)–based therapies, as either single agents or in combination. A retrospective analysis of 1,054 APC patients revealed that 5-FU-based regimens achieved a median OS of 8.8 months, slightly higher than the 7.8 months for gemcitabine-based regimens (HR = 1.244, 95% CI = 1.090–1.419; $P < 0.001$). Importantly, these therapies also demonstrated comparable PFS, suggesting that both regimens are viable alternatives to RT.

In terms of QoL metrics, avoiding RT-related complications such as fatigue, tissue damage and long-term secondary malignancies is crucial. Chemotherapy regimens with manageable side effects allow for better symptom management and improved functional outcomes (Liu et al., 2024). These findings collectively highlight that advanced chemotherapy not only prolongs survival but also preserves QoL, making it a robust option for managing APC while mitigating the risks of RT.

Study 4

The PRIME II trial was a pivotal study examining the feasibility of hormone therapy alone in older women with early-stage breast cancer. The trial enrolled 1,326 women aged 65 years or older with hormone receptor-positive breast cancer who had undergone breast-conserving surgery. Participants were randomized to receive either whole-breast radiotherapy or no radiotherapy, while all received adjuvant endocrine therapy.

After a median follow-up of 5 years, the trial found that the rate of ipsilateral breast tumour recurrence (IBTR) was 1.3% in the radiotherapy group compared to 4.1% in the no-radiotherapy group. Despite this modest increase in local recurrence among those who skipped radiotherapy, there was no significant difference in the 5-year OS rate, which was 93.9% in both groups. Additionally, patients in the no-radiotherapy group reported better QoL, with less fatigue and improved cosmetic outcomes.

The findings suggest that for older women with low-risk, hormone receptor-positive early breast cancer, hormone therapy alone can be a feasible alternative to radiotherapy. This approach offers a favourable balance between reducing treatment burden and maintaining excellent survival outcomes, with minimal impact on recurrence rates (Kunkler et al., 2015).

GLOBAL PERSPECTIVES ON NO-RT

The shift towards personalized treatment paradigms in oncology is increasingly supported by international bodies such as the European Society for Radiotherapy and Oncology (ESTRO) and International Atomic Energy Agency (IAEA), which advocate for less invasive, more targeted therapies, including options that may not involve radiotherapy (NO-RT). This movement aligns with a broader trend in precision oncology, emphasizing tailored treatments based on individual genetic and molecular profiles.

The application of NO-RT strategies has demonstrated significant potential across various tumour types, with several real-world case studies highlighting both successful outcomes and challenges in implementation. One illustrative case is that of non-Hodgkin's lymphoma. In a prospective trial, approximately 55% of patients with asymptomatic non-Hodgkin's lymphoma with a favourable prognosis were managed with a WW strategy, delaying the initiation of conventional therapies for a median duration of 18 months (Mead et al., 1984). This case study underscores how careful patient selection, based on clinical presentation and prognostic factors, can effectively defer the use of RT without compromising patient outcomes.

Another example can be seen in the management of soft tissue sarcoma (STS). In particular, patients with myxoid liposarcomas have been treated successfully with surgery alone, avoiding the potential toxicities associated with radiation. This tailored approach is driven by a better understanding of tumour biology and histological subtype, which has led to more precise treatment strategies (Gronchi, 2015). However, even in STS, the decision to omit RT is not universal; histology and other patient-specific factors play a crucial role in the decision-making process, highlighting the inherent challenges of implementing NO-RT.

In the context of oligometastatic NSCLC, local ablative therapy (LAT) has emerged as an effective treatment alternative to conventional radiation. Studies report a remarkable overall response rate of 95% and a median OS of 32 months in selected patients, emphasizing the potential of NO-RT strategies when combined with targeted interventions (Badellino et al., 2022). Despite these successes, challenges remain, particularly in standardizing patient selection criteria across diverse clinical settings.

The decision-making process for NO-RT is multifaceted, incorporating tumour characteristics, patient health status and emerging clinical data. In non-resectable head and neck tumours, for instance, treatment decisions are influenced by tumour morphology and patient preferences, with ongoing research striving to refine these criteria (Dietz et al., 2005). Overall, while NO-RT strategies offer a promising avenue for reducing treatment burden and improving QoL, they require meticulous patient selection and a nuanced understanding of disease biology to ensure optimal outcomes.

INTERNATIONAL GUIDELINES AND CONSENSUS STATEMENTS—ESTRO AND IAEA INITIATIVES

Organizations such as the ESTRO and the IAEA have been instrumental in shaping global oncology treatment guidelines. Recent recommendations from these bodies highlight the integration of genomic and molecular profiling into treatment planning, enabling the identification of patients who may not require radiotherapy (Barducci et al., 2024). This shift aims to enhance therapeutic outcomes while reducing treatment-related morbidity.

National Oncology Societies

Various national oncology societies are also promoting consensus statements that prioritize personalized medicine. The American Society of Clinical Oncology (ASCO) and the European Society for Medical Oncology (ESMO) have both endorsed risk-adapted strategies that minimize unnecessary interventions. These guidelines advocate for biomarker-driven decision-making, ensuring that radiotherapy is administered only when it offers significant clinical benefit.

The ESTRO and the IAEA promote less invasive treatment modalities, including NO-RT. These international bodies work to standardize radiotherapy practices, improve treatment quality and ensure patient safety across diverse healthcare systems worldwide. Their contributions are particularly impactful in low- and middle-income countries (LMICs), where resource constraints often challenge the delivery of advanced cancer treatments (Thariat et al., 2024).

ESTRO has been at the forefront of developing consensus statements and guidelines that advocate for the adoption of innovative radiotherapy techniques. By conducting extensive surveys and collaborative studies, ESTRO has documented the variability in radiotherapy practices across different regions and has emphasized the need for standardization. For instance, recent surveys assessing re-irradiation practices have highlighted the potential of NO-RT in reducing treatment-related toxicity while maintaining clinical efficacy (Bleaney & Thippu Jayaprakash, 2024). ESTRO's recommendations focus not only on the technical aspects of treatment but also on improving overall patient outcomes through personalized, less invasive approaches.

Similarly, the IAEA plays a critical role in enhancing radiotherapy services globally. Through its quality assurance programs, safety audits and educational initiatives, the IAEA seeks to address disparities in cancer care between high-income and resource-limited settings (Salminen et al., 2005; Lam et al., 2016). The agency's efforts include organizing international workshops and training sessions aimed at upskilling healthcare professionals and promoting evidence-based practices. IAEA initiatives emphasize the importance of integrating new technologies and treatment modalities, such as NO-RT, which have the potential to reduce the adverse effects associated with conventional radiotherapy while ensuring effective tumour control (Abdel-Wahab et al., 2011).

The influence of these international organizations is reflected in evolving practice patterns worldwide. Recent consensus statements encourage the selective omission of radiotherapy in cases where clinical evidence supports a safe de-escalation, thereby reducing patient morbidity and healthcare costs (Rosenblatt et al., 2015). These global initiatives not only foster uniformity in treatment standards but also empower clinicians to tailor therapy based on individual patient profiles, ultimately promoting a more patient-centred approach to cancer care.

GLOBAL TRENDS AND COLLABORATIVE MOVEMENTS—RECENT INTERNATIONAL CLINICAL TRIALS

Several international clinical trials are actively refining patient selection criteria to reduce unnecessary radiotherapy. For example, the PRECISION-RT trial investigated the use of advanced imaging and molecular diagnostics to stratify patients based on their predicted response to radiotherapy, ensuring that only those who truly benefit receive it (Mechahougui et al., 2024). Similarly, the ADAPT-RT study focused on de-escalating radiotherapy in patients with favourable tumour biology, reinforcing the global shift towards individualized care.

IMPACT ON TREATMENT PARADIGMS

The growing emphasis on precision oncology is reshaping traditional cancer treatment approaches. Emerging evidence suggests that targeted therapies, immune checkpoint inhibitors and novel systemic treatments can provide comparable or superior outcomes to radiotherapy in certain patient populations (He et al., 2024). Consequently, NO-RT strategies are gaining traction as viable alternatives, particularly in early-stage and low-risk cancers.

While these advancements hold promise, challenges remain. The accessibility of molecular diagnostics and biomarker testing varies across healthcare systems, potentially limiting the widespread adoption of NO-RT strategies. Additionally, the interpretation of complex genomic data requires robust bioinformatics tools and expertise (Ahmed, 2024). Addressing these barriers is crucial to fully realizing the potential of personalized oncology and optimizing patient care on a global scale.

GOALS

This book is a forward-thinking exploration of cancer treatment strategies that change the traditional reliance on radiation. By the end of this book, readers will possess a deeper understanding of how to integrate NO-RT principles into clinical practice and balance effective cancer management with the preservation of healthy organs and the overall quality of life.

This book starts by defining the NO-RT concept and its increasing relevance to oncology. Here readers will learn the history and evolution of RT and also understand why the medical community is now changing towards the methods or approaches that reduce or avoid radiation when possible. This foundational knowledge can help in framing the discussion that follows. The main aim is to give readers the ability to recognize when NO-RT approaches can be used. This involves having a deeper knowledge of tumour biology, analysis of risk–benefit, biomarker usage and genetic profiling for predicting patient response. From this readers will gain the skills for assessing specific tumour types and identifying when alternative treatments can be useful. Additionally, readers will explore how various treatment modalities like surgery, chemotherapy and other innovative therapies such as ultrasound and immunotherapy can complement the NO-RT approach. This book will show how these alternative methods can provide effective treatment without any potential damage from radiation. The development of a patient-focused approach is significant. This book will outline the criteria for selecting patients who can benefit most from NO-RT by discussing multidisciplinary evaluations and understanding the ethical considerations of withholding radiation. Readers will learn to personalize the treatment plans mainly based on the individual needs of the patients. To connect theory and practice, this book offers decision-making algorithms and clinical pathways to integrate NO-RT into conventional cancer treatment protocols. Personalization and follow-up strategies will be given in detail by highlighting the documentation for tracking the outcomes.

This book includes detailed case studies that provide details of both successful and challenging applications of NO-RT by providing a wide range of real-world scenarios. These case studies will explore the patient outcomes, decision-making processes and factors that contribute to the success or reconsideration of NO-RT. From these case studies, readers can learn the treatment complexities and highlight best practices with practical examples. The challenges in adopting NO-RT are also addressed, including the technological limitations, clinician's mindset and financial implications. By evaluating these challenges, readers can get a realistic perspective on current barriers and promising advancements that may overcome them. Discussions regarding future directions will provide a pathway for ongoing development and integration of NO-RT in clinical practice. This structured approach ensures that by the end of the book, readers will not only understand the concept of NO-RT but also implement and advocate it in oncology.

To dive deeper into when to opt for each approach, **Table 1.1** provides a clearer understanding of how to select the best-suited option for patients, indicating when radiotherapy is essential and when non-radiation therapy could be considered, keeping patient safety in mind.

TABLE 1.1 When RT Is Essential vs. When to Consider NO-RT

Criteria	When RT Is Essential	When to Consider NO-RT
Tumour Biology and Risk	• Aggressive tumour types (e.g., triple-negative breast cancer, high-risk NSCLC)	• Favourable tumour biology (e.g., luminal A breast cancer in older patients)
Patient Demographics	• Younger patients with higher recurrence risk	• Older patients or those with low-risk profiles where toxicity is a concern
Treatment Response and Strategy	• Insufficient response to systemic therapies	• Effective alternative modalities (e.g., advanced chemotherapy, targeted therapies, minimally invasive surgery)
Clinical Evidence	• Clinical trials showing survival benefit and improved local control when RT is administered	• Trials (e.g., PRIME II, OPRA, QUARTZ) demonstrating comparable outcomes with reduced side effects through de-escalation
Quality-of-Life Considerations	• Cases where the aggressive nature of cancer necessitates the benefits of RT despite potential side effects	• Situations where preserving quality of life and minimizing treatment-related morbidity are prioritized

REFERENCES

Abdel-Wahab, M., Rosenblatt, E., Holmberg, O., & Meghzifene, A. (2011). Safety in radiation oncology: The role of international initiatives by the International Atomic Energy Agency. *Journal of the American College of Radiology*, *8*(11), 789–794. https://doi.org/10.1016/j.jacr.2011.07.014

Ahmed, F. J. (2024). Personalized medicine: The dawn of a new era in healthcare. *Futuristic Biotechnology*, 01. https://doi.org/10.54393/fbt.v4i03.138

Badellino, S., Levis, M., Cuffini, E., Cerrato, M., Orlandi, E., Chiovatero, I., Aprile, A., Gastino, A., Cavallin, C., Iorio, G., Parise, R., Mantovani, C., & Ricardi, U. (2022). Role of radiosurgery and stereotactic ablative radiotherapy for oligometastatic non-oncogene addicted NSCLC. *Cancers*, *14*(6), 1465. https://doi.org/10.3390/cancers14061465

Barducci, M. C., Tozzi, V. D., Pelizzari, G., Aprile, G., Grossi, F., Pinto, C., Fasola, G., Regattin, L., Follador, A., Loreto, C. D., Pizzolitto, S., Longanesi, A., Guglielmi, A., Zanconati, F., Toscani, P., Rabusin, M., Trua, N., Franceschi, S., Baldassarre, G., … Sulfaro, S. (2024). Precision oncology implementation in a regional-based health care system: A professional consensus to define the pathway. *Journal of Cancer Policy*, *42*, 100515. https://doi.org/10.1016/j.jcpo.2024.100515

Barton, M. B., Frommer, M., & Shafiq, J. (2006). Role of radiotherapy in cancer control in low-income and middle-income countries. *Lancet Oncology*, *7*(7), 584–595. https://doi.org/10.1016/S1470-2045(06)70759-8

Barton, M. B., Jacob, S., Shafiq, J., Wong, K., Thompson, S. R., Hanna, T. P., & Delaney, G. P. (2014). Estimating the demand for radiotherapy from the evidence: A review of changes from 2003 to 2012. *Radiotherapy and Oncology*, *112*(1), 140–144. https://doi.org/10.1016/j.radonc.2014.03.024

Bernhardt, D., El Shafie, R., Thomas, M., Bozorgmehr, F., Schiele, A., Schmitt, D., Welzel, T., Thalmann, P., Paul, A., König, L., Lang, K., Adeberg, S., Höne, S., Weykamp, F., Vollmuth, P., Lentz-Hommertgen, A., Jaekel, C., Nestle, U., Kieser, M., … Rieken, S. (2023). Stereotactic radiotherapy vs. Whole brain radiation therapy for patients with 1–10 brain metastases from small cell lung cancer: Results of the randomized encephalon (ARO 2018–9) trial. *International Journal of Radiation Oncology*Biology*Physics*, *117*(4), e5. https://doi.org/10.1016/j.ijrobp.2023.08.031

Bleaney, C. W., & Thippu Jayaprakash, K. (2024). Oncoflash—Research updates in a flash. *Clinical Oncology*, *36*(7), 399–401. https://doi.org/10.1016/j.clon.2024.05.009

Buschke, F. (1970). Radiation therapy: The past, the present, the future: Janeway lecture, 1969. *American Journal of Roentgenology*, *108*(2), 236–246. https://doi.org/10.2214/ajr.108.2.236

Cao, B., Zhang, L., Wu, C., Liu, X., Wang, Q., Tong, F., Yang, W., & Wang, J. (2023). Survival outcomes and failure patterns in patients with inoperable non-metastatic pancreatic cancer treated with definitive radiotherapy. *Cancers*, *15*(8), 2213. https://doi.org/10.3390/cancers15082213

Datta, D., Engineer, R., Saklani, A., D'souza, A., Baheti, A., Kumar, S., Krishnatry, R., Ostwal, V., Ramaswamy, A., & Patil, P. (2024). Non-operative management in low-lying rectal cancers undergoing chemoradiation. *Journal of Cancer Research and Therapeutics*, *20*(1), 417–422. https://doi.org/10.4103/jcrt.jcrt_189_23

De Jong, D., Das, J. P., Ma, H., Pailey Valiplackal, J., Prendergast, C., Roa, T., Braumuller, B., Deng, A., Dercle, L., Yeh, R., Salvatore, M. M., & Capaccione, K. M. (2023). Novel targets, novel treatments: The changing landscape of non-small cell lung cancer. *Cancers*, *15*(10), 2855. https://doi.org/10.3390/cancers15102855

De Santis, P., Perrone, M., Guarini, C., Santoro, A. N., Laface, C., Carrozzo, D., Oliva, G. R., & Fedele, P. (2024). Early-stage triple negative breast cancer: The therapeutic role of immunotherapy and the prognostic value of pathological complete response. *Exploration of Targeted Anti-Tumor Therapy*, *5*(1), 232–250. https://doi.org/10.37349/etat.2024.00215

Dietz, A., Weber, A., Dollner, R., & Hildebrandt, G. (2005). Nicht resektable kopf-hals- tumoren und deren therapie. *Laryngo-Rhino-Otologie*, *84*(3), 200–206. https://doi.org/10.1055/s-2005-861132

Goffredo, P., Quezada-Diaz, F. F., Garcia-Aguilar, J., & Smith, J. J. (2022). Non-operative management of patients with rectal cancer: Lessons learnt from the OPRA trial. *Cancers*, *14*(13), 3204. https://doi.org/10.3390/cancers14133204

Gospodarowicz, M., Trypuc, J., D'Cruz, A., Khader, J., Omar, S., & Knaul, F. (2015). Cancer services and the comprehensive cancer center. In H. Gelband, P. Jha, R. Sankaranarayanan & S. Horton (Eds.), *Cancer: Disease Control Priorities*, Third Edition (Volume 3). The International Bank for Reconstruction and Development/The World Bank. http://www.ncbi.nlm.nih.gov/books/NBK343637/

Gresham, G. K., Wells, G. A., Gill, S., Cameron, C., & Jonker, D. J. (2014). Chemotherapy regimens for advanced pancreatic cancer: A systematic review and network meta-analysis. *BMC Cancer*, *14*(1), 471. https://doi.org/10.1186/1471-2407-14-471

Gronchi, A. (2015). Individualizing the use/non-use of radiation therapy (RT) in soft tissue sarcoma (STS): When abstention is better than care: Individualizing the use/non-use of radiation therapy. *Journal of Surgical Oncology*, *111*(2), 133–134. https://doi.org/10.1002/jso.23827

Hamdy, F. C., Donovan, J. L., Lane, J. A., Mason, M., Metcalfe, C., Holding, P., Davis, M., Peters, T. J., Turner, E. L., Martin, R. M., Oxley, J., Robinson, M., Staffurth, J., Walsh, E., Bollina, P., Catto, J., Doble, A., Doherty, A., Gillatt, D., … ProtecT Study Group. (2016). 10-year outcomes after monitoring, surgery, or radiotherapy for localized prostate cancer. *New England Journal of Medicine*, *375*(15), 1415–1424. https://doi.org/10.1056/NEJMoa1606220

He, W., McCoy, M. D., Riggins, R. B., Beckman, R. A., & Yeang, C.-H. (2024). Personalized cancer treatment strategies incorporating irreversible and reversible drug resistance mechanisms. *NPJ Systems Biology and Applications*, *11*(1), 70. https://doi.org/10.1101/2024.11.03.621749

Holsti, L. R. (1995). Development of clinical radiotherapy since 1896. *Acta Oncologica*, *34*(8), 995–1003. https://doi.org/10.3109/02841869509127225

Hughes, K. S., Schnaper, L. A., Bellon, J. R., Cirrincione, C. T., Berry, D. A., McCormick, B., Muss, H. B., Smith, B. L., Hudis, C. A., Winer, E. P., & Wood, W. C. (2013). Lumpectomy plus tamoxifen with or without irradiation in women age 70 years or older with early breast cancer: Long-term follow-up of CALGB 9343. *Journal of Clinical Oncology*, *31*(19), 2382–2387. https://doi.org/10.1200/JCO.2012.45.2615

Huh, H. D., & Kim, S (2020). History of radiation therapy technology. *Progress in Medical Physics*, *31*(3), 124–134. https://doi.org/10.14316/pmp.2020.31.3.124

Imlach, F., Dunn, A., Costello, S., Gurney, J., & Sarfati, D. (2023). Driving quality improvement through better data: The story of New Zealand's radiation oncology collection. *Journal of Medical Imaging and Radiation Oncology*, *67*(1), 119–127. https://doi.org/10.1111/1754-9485.13488

Jaffray, D. A., & Gospodarowicz, M. K. (2015). Radiation therapy for cancer. In H. Gelband, P. Jha, R. Sankaranarayanan & S. Horton (Eds.), *Cancer: Disease Control Priorities*, Third Edition (Volume 3). The International Bank for Reconstruction and Development/The World Bank. http://www.ncbi.nlm.nih.gov/books/NBK343621/

Kunkler, I. H., Williams, L. J., Jack, W. J. L., Cameron, D. A., & Dixon, J. M. (2015). Breast-conserving surgery with or without irradiation in women aged 65 years or older with early breast cancer (PRIME ii): A randomised controlled trial. *Lancet Oncology*, *16*(3), 266–273. https://doi.org/10.1016/S1470-2045(14)71221-5

Lam, K.-O., Lee, A. W. M., Ng, W.-T., & Hopkins, K. I. (2016). The International Atomic Energy Agency global initiatives on nasopharyngeal cancer treatment. *Chinese Clinical Oncology*, *5*(2), 27. https://doi.org/10.21037/cco.2016.03.02

Lederman, M. (1981). The early history of radiotherapy: 1895–1939. *International Journal of Radiation Oncology*Biology*Physics*, *7*(5), 639–648. https://doi.org/10.1016/0360-3016(81)90379-5

Liu, S.-Y. M., Zheng, M.-M., Pan, Y., Liu, S.-Y., Li, Y., & Wu, Y.-L. (2023). Emerging evidence and treatment paradigm of non-small cell lung cancer. *Journal of Hematology & Oncology*, *16*(1), 40. https://doi.org/10.1186/s13045-023-01436-2

Liu, Y., Guo, X., Xu, P., Song, Y., Huang, J., Chen, X., Zhu, W., Hao, J., & Gao, S. (2024). Clinical outcomes of second-line chemotherapy in patients with advanced pancreatic adenocarcinoma: A real-world study. *Cancer Biology & Medicine*, 1–14. https://doi.org/10.20892/j.issn.2095-3941.2024.0036

Mead, G. M., Macbeth, F. R., Ryall, R. D. H., Williams, C. J., & Whitehouse, J. M. A. (1984). A report on a prospective trial of no initial therapy in patients with asymptomatic favourable prognosis non-Hodgkin's lymphoma. *Hematological Oncology, 2*(2), 179–188. https://doi.org/10.1002/hon.2900020207

Mechahougui, H., Gutmans, J., Colarusso, G., Gouasmi, R., & Friedlaender, A. (2024). Advances in personalized oncology. *Cancers, 16*(16), 2862. https://doi.org/10.3390/cancers16162862

Ng, I. W., Tey, J. C. S., Chia, D. W. T., Yee, C. M., & Cheo, T. S. T. (2019). A review of whole brain radiotherapy outcomes in a high epidermal growth factor receptor mutation rate population: Does QUARTZ apply in Asia? *Asia-Pacific Journal of Clinical Oncology, 15*(6), 353–357. https://doi.org/10.1111/ajco.13223

Nieder, C., Dalhaug, A., & Pawinski, A. (2020). Confirmatory analysis of quartz study results: Survival prolongation after whole-brain radiotherapy. *Anticancer Research, 40*(2), 977–981. https://doi.org/10.21873/anticanres.14031

Premnath, N., & Madanat, Y. F. (2023). Paradigm shift in the management of acute myeloid leukemia—Approved options in 2023. *Cancers, 15*(11), 3002. https://doi.org/10.3390/cancers15113002

Rosenblatt, E., Acuña, O., & Abdel-Wahab, M. (2015). The challenge of global radiation therapy: An IAEA perspective. *International Journal of Radiation Oncology*Biology*Physics, 91*(4), 687–689. https://doi.org/10.1016/j.ijrobp.2014.12.008

Salminen, E., Izewska, J., & Andreo, P. (2005). IAEA's role in the global management of cancer—Focus on upgrading radiotherapy services. *Acta Oncologica, 44*(8), 816–824. https://doi.org/10.1080/02841860500341355

Smith, J. J., Chow, O. S., Gollub, M. J., Nash, G. M., Temple, L. K., Weiser, M. R., Guillem, J. G., Paty, P. B., Avila, K., & Garcia-Aguilar, J. (2015). Organ preservation in rectal adenocarcinoma: A phase II randomized controlled trial evaluating 3-year disease-free survival in patients with locally advanced rectal cancer treated with chemoradiation plus induction or consolidation chemotherapy, and total mesorectal excision or nonoperative management. *BMC Cancer, 15*(1), 767. https://doi.org/10.1186/s12885-015-1632-z

Starkey, D. E., Bhatnagar, D. A., Bates, D. A., Fenton, D. P., Wood, D. V., Begum, M. N., & Main, D. S. (2024). Whole brain radiotherapy for intracranial metastatic disease in non-small cell lung cancer: The Wessex experience. *Neuro-Oncology, 26*(Supplement_7), vii13. https://doi.org/10.1093/neuonc/noae158.051

Thames, H. D. (1988). Early fractionation methods and the origins of the NSD concept. *Acta Oncologica, 27*(2), 89–103. https://doi.org/10.3109/02841868809090329

Thariat, J., Little, M. P., Zablotska, L. B., Samson, P., O'Banion, M. K., Leuraud, K., Bergom, C., Girault, G., Azimzadeh, O., Bouffler, S., & Hamada, N. (2024). Radiotherapy for non-cancer diseases: Benefits and long-term risks. *International Journal of Radiation Biology, 100*(4), 505–526. https://doi.org/10.1080/09553002.2023.2295966

Thompson, H. M., Omer, D. M., Lin, S., Kim, J. K., Yuval, J. B., Verheij, F. S., Qin, L.- X., Gollub, M. J., Wu, A. J.-C., Lee, M., Patil, S., Hezel, A. F., Marcet, J. E., Cataldo, P. A., Polite, B. N., Herzig, D. O., Liska, D., Oommen, S., Friel, C. M., … OPRA Consortium. (2024). Organ preservation and survival by clinical response grade in patients with rectal cancer treated with total neoadjuvant therapy: A secondary analysis of the OPRA randomized clinical trial. *JAMA Network Open, 7*(1), e2350903. https://doi.org/10.1001/jamanetworkopen.2023.50903

Trikhirhisthit, K., Setakornnukul, J., & Thephamongkhol, K. (2022). Added survival benefit of whole brain radiotherapy in brain metastatic non-small cell lung cancer: Development and external validation of an individual prediction model. *Frontiers in Oncology, 12*, 911835. https://doi.org/10.3389/fonc.2022.911835

Turgeman, I., & Ben-Aharon, I. (2021). Evolving treatment paradigms in esophageal cancer. *Annals of Translational Medicine, 9*(10), 903–903. https://doi.org/10.21037/atm.2020.03.110

Turner, J. H (2024). Theranostic innovation by humane N-of-one cancer care in real-world patients. *Cancer Biotherapy and Radiopharmaceuticals, 39*(5), 323–329. https://doi.org/10.1089/cbr.2023.0198

Tyldesley, S., Delaney, G., Foroudi, F., Barbera, L., Kerba, M., & Mackillop, W. (2011). Estimating the need for radiotherapy for patients with prostate, breast, and lung cancers: Verification of model estimates of need with radiotherapy utilization data from British Columbia. *International Journal of Radiation Oncology*Biology*Physics*, *79*(5), 1507–1515. https://doi.org/10.1016/j.ijrobp.2009.12.070

Whelan, T. J., Smith, S., Parpia, S., Fyles, A. W., Bane, A., Liu, F.-F., Rakovitch, E., Chang, L., Stevens, C., Bowen, J., Provencher, S., Théberge, V., Mulligan, A. M., Kos, Z., Akra, M. A., Voduc, K. D., Hijal, T., Dayes, I. S., Pond, G., … Levine, M. N. (2023). Omitting radiotherapy after breast-conserving surgery in luminal a breast cancer. *New England Journal of Medicine*, *389*(7), 612–619. https://doi.org/10.1056/NEJMoa2302344

Wolf, A. S. (2023). Commentary: Nothing is free: Surgeons' and radiation oncologists' biases about treating early-stage lung cancer in healthy patients. *Journal of Thoracic and Cardiovascular Surgery*, S0022522323009868. https://doi.org/10.1016/j.jtcvs.2023.10.029

Wong, C. H. L., Kam, T. Y., Fong, J. K. S., Lee, V. H. F., Chiu, M. K. L., Cheung, K. M., Nyaw, S. F., Lim, M. Y., Kwan, C. K., Mok, S. T. F., & Lee, A. W. M. (2024). 175P Quality of life in patients with NSCLC brain metastases undergoing different local therapies in the era of precision oncology: A territory-wide study. *ESMO Open*, *9*(Suppl S3), Article 102905. https://doi.org/10.1016/j.esmoop.2024.102905

CHAPTER 2

Recognizing Tumour Biology and Assessing Radiation Therapy Need

Mangesh Korde and Mukesh Chandra

INTRODUCTION

Understanding tumour biology is significant in modern oncology mainly when the need for radiation therapy is considered. The decision-making process mostly involves the evaluation of tumour characteristics, patient-specific factors and emerging scientific data. Tumour characteristics such as growth rate, molecular profile and potential for metastasis are significant factors in the development of appropriate treatment strategies. This chapter explains how these biological factors influence the decisions to use or avoid radiation therapy (RT). It discusses the critical balance of risk and benefits for determining the proper RT use by taking patient health and tumour location into consideration.

Biomarkers and genetic profiling are considered essential tools for predicting the tumour response to RT and helping in personalized treatment plans. These molecular markers will help in more precise therapeutic decisions by reducing unnecessary radiation exposure and optimizing the outcomes. Specific tumour types, mainly in certain early stages and low-risk cancers, are assessed for their suitability for no radiation therapy (NO-RT) approaches. Conditions such as early-stage hormone receptor-positive breast cancer or well-differentiated thyroid cancers can be considered as examples where RT can be avoided sometimes.

This chapter also provides real-world case studies that help illustrate the successful applications of NO-RT protocols. This shows the influence of tumour biology on the choice of treatment and the move towards more personalized and patient-centred care.

INFLUENCE OF TUMOUR BIOLOGY ON NO-RT DECISIONS

The decision to implement or forgo RT is increasingly driven by the intricate details of tumour biology, which includes factors such as PD-L1 expression, tumour hypoxia, size and genetic mutations. Personalized treatment plans that incorporate these factors can significantly optimize outcomes by determining when RT can be safely avoided and when it remains necessary.

DOI: 10.1201/9781003529071-2

For instance, lung tumours exhibiting high PD-L1 expression (≥50%) have been shown to respond favourably to immunotherapy. In such cases, the robust immune response elicited by these agents may negate the need for RT, as seen in metastatic non-small cell lung cancer (NSCLC) where patients with high PD-L1 levels experienced improved survival outcomes when treated solely with immunotherapy (Moran et al., 2022; Smith et al., 2024). Conversely, tumours characterized by hypoxia often present challenges for systemic therapies due to limited drug penetration. In these scenarios, RT can be particularly effective in overcoming the hypoxic barrier by directly damaging the tumour's DNA, thereby complementing systemic treatment strategies. **Figure 2.1** provides a decision-making algorithm for radiotherapy (RT) versus NO-RT approaches. The flowchart outlines a tumour biology-driven framework for treatment selection. Factors such as PD-L1 expression, hypoxia status, tumour size and biomarker profiles guide whether patients may benefit from immunotherapy, hypoxia-targeting agents, multimodal approaches including RT or selective omission of RT (NO-RT). Standard RT protocols remain the default in the absence of favourable biomarker profiles.

Additionally, tumour size plays a critical role in treatment decisions. Larger tumours, generally those exceeding 5 cm, often correlate with a higher disease burden and may benefit from a multimodal approach that includes RT, especially when rapid local control is necessary (Smith et al., 2024). Patient comorbidities also factor into this decision-making process; individuals with significant health challenges might be steered towards less aggressive treatments, emphasizing the need for tailored approaches.

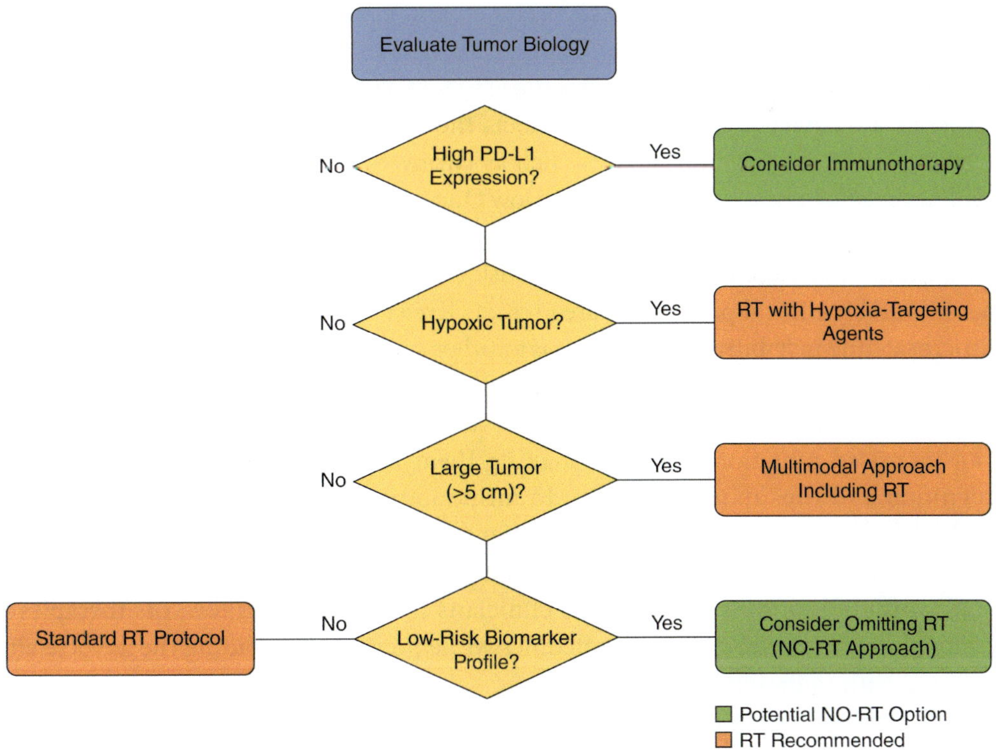

FIGURE 2.1 Decision-making flowchart based on tumour biology.

Genetic mutations further complicate the landscape. For example, tumours harbouring *EGFR* mutations alongside high PD-L1 expression may exhibit variable responses to targeted therapies alone, suggesting that RT might still be needed for optimal local control (Moran et al., 2022). Thus, the integration of molecular profiling and tumour biology is essential in guiding clinicians towards personalized, evidence-based decisions regarding the use of RT versus alternative treatment modalities.

BIOMARKERS

Biomarkers have emerged as critical tools in personalizing cancer treatment, particularly when it comes to determining whether RT can be safely omitted. These biomarkers provide valuable insights into tumour biology, patient prognosis and potential treatment responses, allowing clinicians to tailor therapeutic strategies to individual patient needs.

One of the most notable biomarkers is the Decipher genomic score, used predominantly in prostate cancer management. The Decipher score is derived from the analysis of gene expression profiles obtained from prostate cancer tissue samples. By examining the activity of multiple genes associated with cancer progression and metastasis, the Decipher assay categorizes patients into different risk groups. Patients with low Decipher scores have a reduced likelihood of metastasis and disease progression. As a result, these patients may be considered for a less aggressive treatment approach, including the omission of RT following surgery. By identifying individuals who are at low risk of recurrence, the Decipher score not only minimizes exposure to the potential side effects of RT but also supports a more cost-effective treatment paradigm (Herlemann et al., 2019; Sutera et al., 2022).

In the realm of breast cancer, the Oncotype DX assay serves a similar purpose in refining treatment decisions. This assay evaluates the expression of 21 genes within the tumour tissue to generate a recurrence score, which predicts the likelihood of cancer recurrence and the potential benefit of adjuvant therapies such as chemotherapy. For patients with early-stage hormone receptor-positive breast cancer, a low Oncotype DX score suggests that the addition of systemic therapies may offer minimal benefit. In such cases, the risk of overtreatment is reduced, and these patients might also be considered for an NO-RT approach, particularly if other favourable clinical parameters are present (Kretschmer & Tilki, 2017).

Microsatellite instability (MSI) status is another crucial biomarker, especially in colorectal cancer. MSI refers to the presence of genetic hypermutability that results from defects in the DNA mismatch repair system. Tumours with high MSI (MSI-H) are characterized by an increased mutational burden, making them more susceptible to immune system recognition and thus more responsive to immunotherapy. In colorectal cancer, patients with MSI-H tumours often demonstrate better responses to immune checkpoint inhibitors (ICIs), which can serve as an effective alternative to conventional treatments, including RT. The identification of MSI status allows clinicians to steer patients towards therapies that are more likely to yield favourable outcomes while potentially avoiding the adverse effects associated with radiation (Le et al., 2017).

While the integration of biomarkers like Decipher, Oncotype DX and MSI status has revolutionized personalized oncology, challenges remain regarding their widespread clinical adoption. Continuous research is necessary to validate these biomarkers further and to integrate additional molecular data into treatment decision algorithms. However, the current evidence strongly supports the use of these assays to identify patients who might safely forego RT, thereby reducing unnecessary treatment-related morbidity and improving overall patient quality of life.

By harnessing the power of genomic and molecular biomarkers, clinicians are now better equipped to make nuanced treatment decisions. These tools facilitate the development of personalized treatment plans that optimize efficacy while minimizing exposure to the potential toxicities of RT, marking a significant step forward in the era of precision oncology.

UNDERSTANDING TUMOUR BIOLOGY

Having a complete knowledge of the characteristics of tumours is important for effective treatment strategies in oncology. Tumours exhibit some unique features such as genetic mutation, microenvironmental conditions and evasion from the immune system. These all may affect the treatment decisions significantly. This detail helps in the development of targeted therapies that can improve patient outcomes.

TUMOUR MICROENVIRONMENT AND TREATMENT RESPONSE

The tumour microenvironment (TME) significantly influences treatment response by playing an important role in the efficacy of chemotherapy and immunotherapy. Complex interactions within the TME can either improve or reduce the therapeutic effectiveness. This provides the importance of understanding these functions and metabolisms for optimizing treatment approaches as shown in **Figure 2.2**.

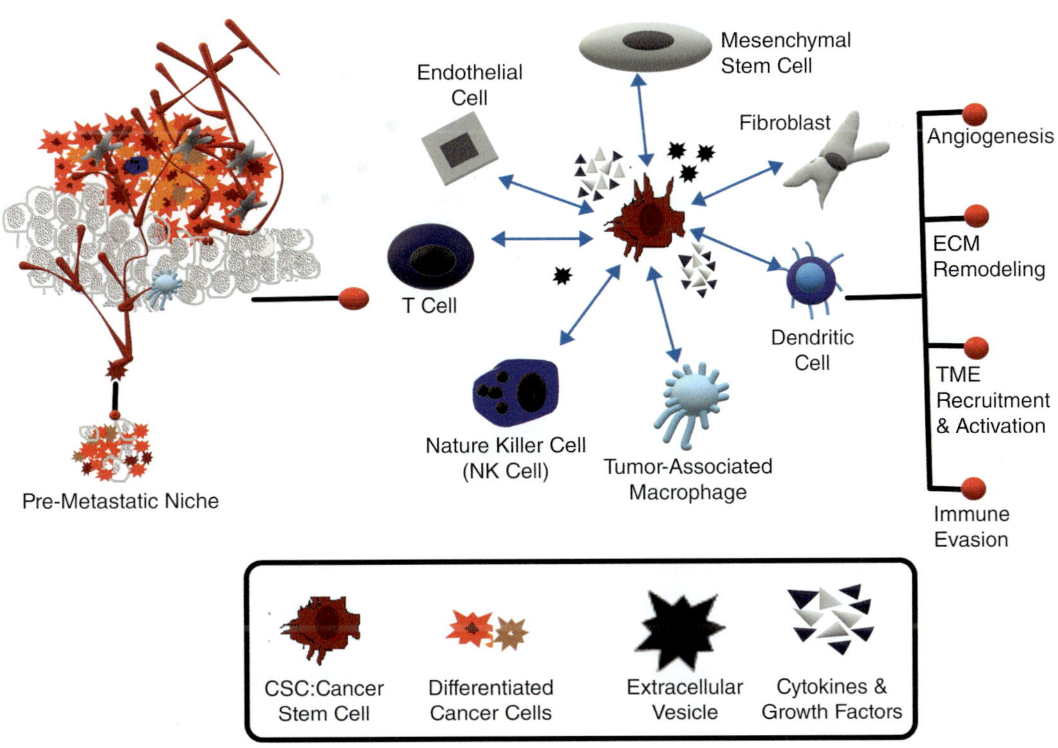

FIGURE 2.2 Interaction of cancer stem cells (CSCs) with the tumour microenvironment.

The tumour often has a distinct microenvironment that can affect the air behaviour and treatment response. For example, hypoxia, which involves slow oxygen levels and acidic conditions, is more prevalent in many solid tumours, and it contributes to the resistance against the conventional therapies that include chemotherapy and radiation. The hypoxic environment reduces RT that mainly relies on oxygen for creating reactive oxygen species that can damage the tumour DNA. Also, an acidic extracellular environment can change drug transportation and cause deficiency by limiting the effectiveness of the chemotherapeutic agent (Jia et al., 2024). The TME is mainly composed of a variety of cellular constituents that include stromal cells and immune cells that can influence the outcomes of treatment. Myeloid cells and cancer-associated fibroblasts have been related to the chemotherapy response in breast cancer, as they act as predictive markers for the success of the treatment (Dhruba et al., 2024). Their presence can support or inhibit cancer progression mainly based on the signals that they produce within the TME. Biochemical alterations such as acidic pH and hypoxia are prevalent in various tumours and contribute to resistance to treatments. For example, hypoxia helps in cancer cell survival by stabilizing the hypoxia-inducible factors that help in promoting angiogenesis and metabolic reprogramming, making the treatment less effective (Wang et al., 2023). Components and interactions within the tumour microenvironment. The schematic depicts the role of various cellular and molecular components in shaping the tumour microenvironment. Tumour cells interact with cancer-associated fibroblasts (CAFs), tumour-associated macrophages (TAMs), TILs/Tregs, and neighbouring stromal cells to promote tumour proliferation, immune evasion, and extracellular matrix (ECM) remodelling. Growth factors (e.g., VEGF, HGF, EGF), cytokines (e.g., IL-6, IL-8, IL-1), chemokines and matrix metalloproteinases (MMPs) further enhance angiogenesis, invasion, epithelial–mesenchymal transition (EMT) and chronic inflammation, collectively driving tumour progression (see **Figure 2.3**).

Some of the approaches, like inhibition of angiogenesis or usage of ICIs aimed at TME modulation, have shown some potential for patient outcome improvement. These interventions try to create an environment that is favourable for therapeutic agents to act on tumours (Goenka et al., 2023; Wang et al., 2023). Advanced delivery systems are another approach that was developed to respond to the TME conditions. The pH-sensitive hydrogels have improved the efficacy of chemotherapy by ensuring the targeted release of drugs at the tumour site (Kim et al., 2023).

GENETIC AND MOLECULAR CHARACTERISTICS

The genetic and molecular characteristics of tumours are critical for understanding their behaviour, treatment responses and progression. Some of the common features include high rates of proliferation, apoptosis dysregulation and evasion of the immune system that may result from alterations in genes impacting the key signalling pathways (Cooper, 2000). One of the examples is that alterations in pathways like PI3K/AKT and RAS/ERK may lead to unchecked cell growth and survival, in which the target therapy inhibit these pathways to be effective (Glaviano et al., 2023). The inhibitors targeting these pathways such as P13K inhibitors are more effective in treating the tumours that have aberrant

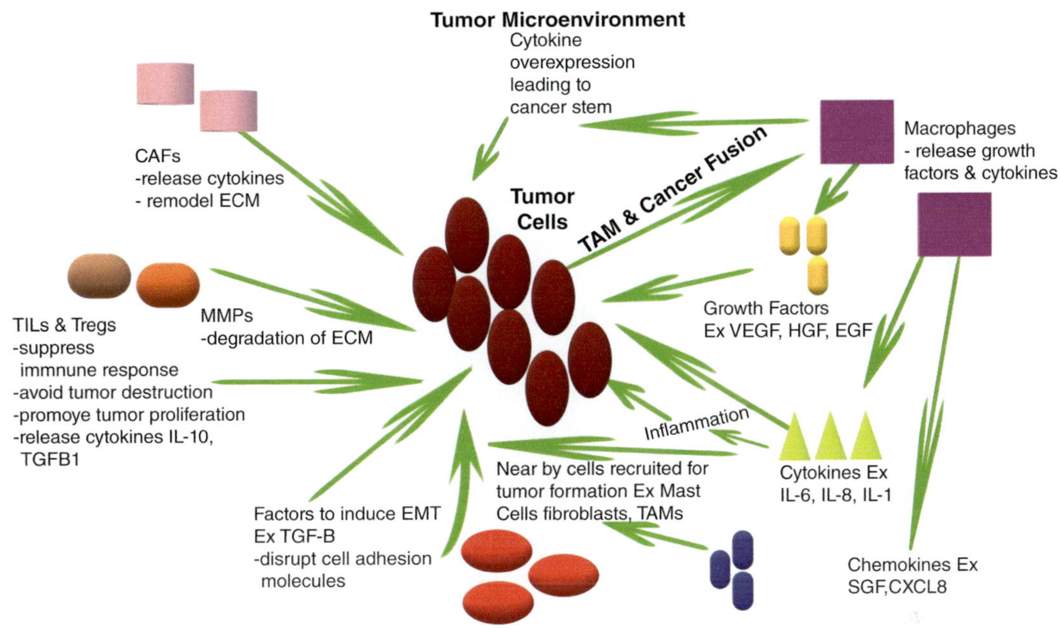

FIGURE 2.3 Generalized model of tumour microenvironment interactions: roles of non-cancerous cells. (CAFs, Cancer-associated fibroblasts; TAMs, Tumour-associated macrophages; TILs, Tumour-infiltrating lymphocytes; Tregs, Regulatory T-cells.)

pathway activation (He et al., 2021). Specific mutations such as overexpression of HER-2 in breast cancer or *K-ras* mutations in colorectal cancer may act as predictive markers for targeted therapy (Valentini et al., 2018).

Certain genetic variations are linked to aggressive tumour behaviour. For example, pathogenic mutations in genes like *BRCA1/2* increase the risk of cancer and also influence tumour progression and response to treatment. Genetic screening for the variants is significant for proper patient selection for targeted treatments. This allows for more personalized and effective care for patients with certain tumours (Petrucelli et al., 1993). Also studied are exceptional responders, that is, the patient who will respond extraordinarily well to the treatments. It is observed that patients have a unique molecular profile, like a proficient DNA damage response mechanism and engagement of the immune system. This leads to exceptional outcomes, and this can help in the development of therapies using similar pathways (Glaviano et al., 2023). Increased genomic stability and structural variations can be used to identify metastatic tumours. The instability of the genome will affect treatment planning because it affects the tumour mechanism and response to the therapies (Ferguson et al., 2015).

EVOLUTION AND HETEROGENEITY OF TUMOURS

The evolution and heterogeneity of tumours are significant factors that can influence the progression of the cancer and the outcomes of the treatment. Tumours show significant genetic diversity starting from mechanisms like chromosomal rearrangement, clonal evolution and environmental factors. Understanding this process is important for providing an effective therapeutic strategy.

Alterations in the chromosomes, including the translocations and the copy number variations, are often observed in tumour evolution, and they can disturb the tumour suppressor genes. In melanoma, some rearrangements affect *NF1* and *CDKN2A*. This affects the growth of tumours and response to treatment. Some advanced analytical methods like HiDENSEC can help in providing a detailed analysis of these rearrangements and provide details regarding the complex structure in heterogeneous tumours (Erdmann-Pham et al., 2023). The relationship between the genomic heterogeneity and immune heterogeneity in the primary tumours and metastasis can be complex. In research on lung cancer, metastasis to the brain has shown that metastasis may need distinct genetic features that differ from the primary tumours. This variability means it is necessary to obtain a personalized treatment method that is made for a unique profile of each tumour (Chen et al., 2023). Even within a single tumour, the heterogeneity may lead to resistance to treatment. Studies regarding meningiomas have identified that differences in genetic expression profiles within the tumours can result from clonal evolution, and it will complicate the treatment outcome. In addition, the special distribution of the subclonal variance may also lead to this complexity, making it challenging to effectively target the tumour cells (Magill et al., 2020). In carcinoma, the tumour heterogeneity is caused by genetic mutation as well as non-genetic changes like epithelial-to-mesenchymal transition (EMT). This shows that environmental factors can also significantly contribute to tumour evolution (Zhang et al., 2024). This interaction of genetic and environmental factors causes another type of complexity in the treatment of cancer.

PATIENT SCENARIO 1—HYPOXIC TUMOUR RESPONSE

A patient with locally advanced lung cancer exhibits a hypoxic TME, leading to resistance against standard RT. Hypoxia-targeting agents or increased RT dosage may be considered to improve treatment response. Hypoxia is a key biomarker in lung cancer but lacks integration into clinical guidelines. Advanced detection methods, such as positron emission tomography (PET) imaging and circulating markers offer potential for personalized treatment (Tumor Microenvironment, n.d.). Understanding hypoxia's role could improve prognosis, guide adjuvant therapy decisions and refine NSCLC management, ultimately enhancing patient outcomes (Ancel et al., 2021). **Figure 2.4** illustrates tumour microenvironment and immune cell interactions, showing the complex interplay between tumour cells, effector immune cells, antigen-presenting cells and immunosuppressive cells within the tumour microenvironment. Tumour-mediated mechanisms such as hypoxia, angiogenesis and cytokine release influence immune evasion by suppressing effector cells (NK, NK-T, T cells) and promoting immunosuppressive populations (Tregs, MDSCs, M2-TAMs), thereby facilitating tumour progression.

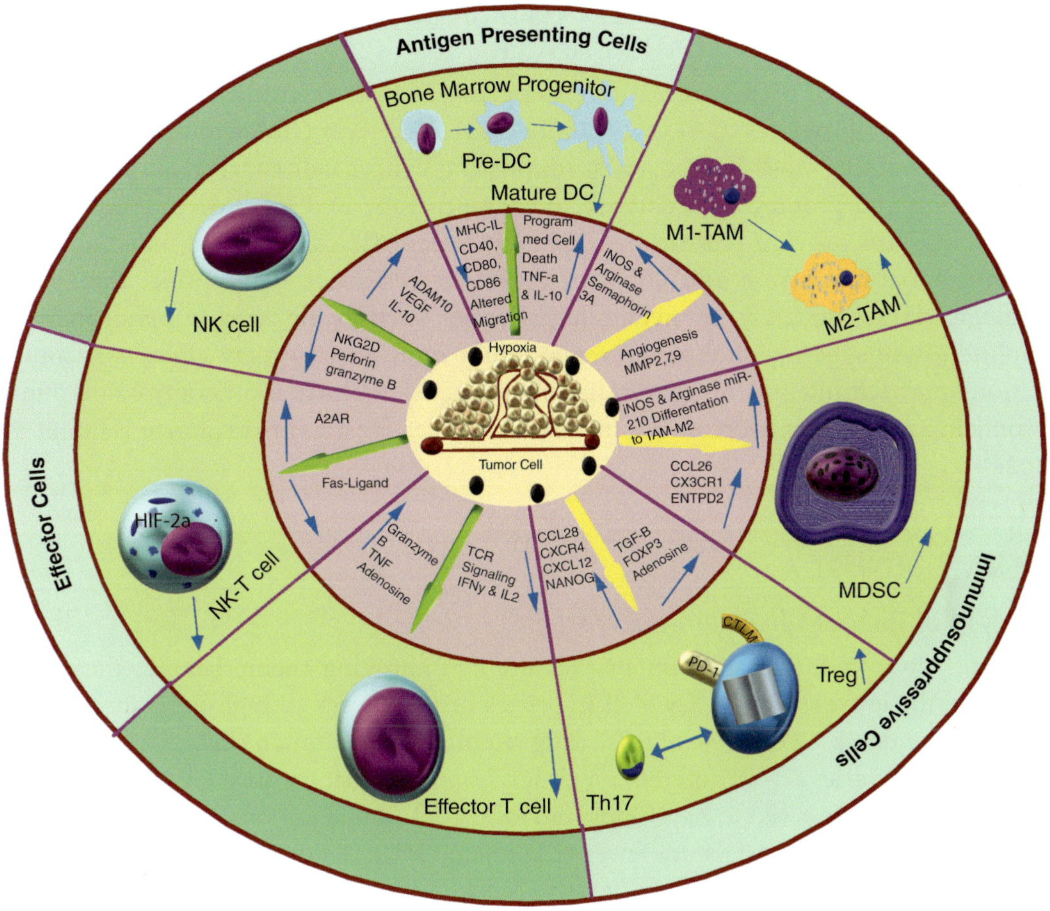

FIGURE 2.4 Graphical overview of hypoxia-induced modulation of immune cells in the tumour microenvironment.

PATIENT SCENARIO 2—IMMUNE CELL INTERACTION

In a patient with triple-negative breast cancer (TNBC) exhibiting immune-suppressive myeloid cells within the TME, the decision to incorporate immunotherapy alongside RT is critical. The presence of myeloid-derived suppressor cells (MDSCs) may hinder the efficacy of RT, prompting the need for strategies to modulate the immune response. The treatment plan could involve administering ICIs to counteract immune suppression, potentially in combination with chemotherapy to enhance T-cell activation and infiltration. Moreover, utilizing agents that target MDSCs or improve dendritic cell function could further optimize the TME, fostering a more favourable environment for RT and immunotherapy synergy. Continuous monitoring of biomarkers related to the TME could guide treatment adjustments, ensuring a personalized approach to therapy that seeks to maximize patient outcomes (Li et al., 2023).

PATIENT SCENARIO 3—CANCER-ASSOCIATED FIBROBLASTS IN PANCREATIC CANCER

A patient diagnosed with pancreatic cancer presents with a significant presence of cancer-associated fibroblasts (CAFs) within the TME. CAFs contribute to tumour progression by sustaining lipid homeostasis, supporting cancer cell survival under nutrient deprivation and promoting resistance to chemotherapy and RT. Recent studies highlight that CAFs provide unsaturated lipids to pancreatic cancer cells, reducing endoplasmic reticulum stress and enhancing tumour resilience. Given this, therapeutic strategies targeting CAFs or metabolic pathways, such as blocking lysophosphatidylcholine-to-phosphatidylcholine conversion, may improve treatment efficacy. A combination approach integrating CAF-targeting therapies with chemotherapy could offer a promising avenue for overcoming pancreatic cancer treatment resistance (Han et al., 2024).

RISK VS. BENEFIT

Analysis of Tumour Characteristics

RT can help in reducing the tumour pressure by improving chemotherapy efficacy. For example, the low-dose RT (1 Gy × 2) improves drug delivery in high-pressure tumours, while higher doses (12 Gy × 3) increase drug retention (Barsoumian et al., 2023). The effectiveness of RT varies across different types. For example, postoperative RT for oesophageal cancer has been observed to have improved local control and survival benefits even if the randomized controlled trials are fewer (Kleinberg, 2010). RT is significant for high-risk ductal carcinoma in situ (DCIS) patients to reduce its recurrence. Also, low-risk patients may avoid RT without compromising outcomes (Smith, 2016).

Long-Term Risks of Radiation Therapy

Despite its benefits, RT causes long-term risks such as second cancer development. Proton beam radiotherapy (PBRT) provides a lower risk of secondary cancers compared to intensity-modulated radiotherapy (IMRT) and three-dimensional conformal radiotherapy (3DCRT) (Xiang et al., 2020). It is crucial to balance the uses of RT and long-term risks. These risks mean it is necessary to plan personalized treatment that helps in balancing uses as well as potential harm.

Benefits of Radiation Therapy

RT provides a curative potential that helps significantly improve survival rates for various cancers. Approximately 3.5 million patients benefit annually from curative treatments. In addition, in advanced cancer cases, RT plays a vital role in palliative care by decreasing symptoms and enhancing quality of life (Bennett, 2021). Some technological improvements such as IMRT and stereotactic body radiotherapy (SBRT) improve precision by decreasing the collateral damage to any healthy tissues and also improve efficacy (LaRiviere & Vapiwala, 2024).

Risks Associated with Radiation Therapy

Despite its benefits, RT has risks, including damage to surrounding healthy tissues, which shows the importance of precisely calculating the dosage (Bennett, 2021). For example, in a study of 152 patients with primary invasive vaginal carcinoma 13.8% experienced late complications that included severe conditions such as rectovaginal fistulas (Blecharz et al., 2013). Head and neck cancer patients undergoing RT frequently suffer from oral morbidities like mucositis and sensory dysfunction, which detrimentally affect the quality of life (Sroussi et al., 2017). Urological complications, including haemorrhagic cystitis and urinary fistulae, present further challenges and can be life-threatening (Chorbińska et al., 2021). Long-term complications such as lung fibrosis have been observed, especially in high-risk breast cancer patients undergoing postmastectomy radiation (Cheng et al., 1998). Furthermore, cost considerations means evaluating the cost risk–benefit analysis to balance financial and health implications (Moores, 2016).

BIOMARKERS AND GENETIC PROFILING

Machine Learning for Biomarker Discovery

By analysing gene expression data that are complex, machine learning (ML) has been used in the discovery of biomarkers. Important genes like *CDKN1A* and *GrIA3* are found using ML. This has classified the radiation dose groups and types of tissues effectively and also with a high precision of $R^2 = 0.97–0.99$ (Andersson et al., 2023). These findings help in the predictive modelling of patient-specific RT responses by advancing precision medicine. Moreover, ML applications also help in imaging biomarkers, where deep learning models extract predictive features from pre-treatment images, assessing causal relationships that guide radiation decisions (Xiao et al., 2024). The tumour behaviour can be obtained with the help of the details given by imaging biomarkers. This may help clinicians in creating personalized treatment plans. By combining the multi-omics datasets, the robustness of biomarker identification can be increased. In this approach, the data related to proteomics, genomics and transcriptomics are combined to predict the response to radiation more accurately. This is similar to the goals of precision medicine (Mathema et al., 2023). Also, the molecular signatures that are identified by ML algorithms support development of personalized cancer therapies as well as improve efficacy and reduce side effects (William et al., 2023).

Germline Genetic Biomarkers

Germline genetic biomarkers are significant in improving personalized medicine in oncology. Some biomarkers such as single-nucleotide polymorphisms (SNPs) and short tandem repeats (STRs) help in the prediction of RT responses. This leads to optimization of treatment strategies and also improves the patient's outcome. Germline variants that are associated with hereditary cancers may have some predictive values for cancer risk. One study has identified that 276 SNPs are related to important cancer pathways. It also discusses their usage in the identification of cancer susceptibility and helping in preventative measures (Dalfovo et al., 2024). These markers will assist in risk stratification as well as improve the treatment planning precision.

By combining the germline biomarkers into clinical oncology, RT can be transformed with accurate decision-making. A study of the Indian population identified 34 germline variants across various cancers that show their potential to provide therapies to individual genetic profiles. Also, these biomarkers act as a diagnostic tool and provide accurate results in the determination of correct treatment modalities (Vatsyayan & Scaria, 2023). Germline genetic variants are related to toxicity and therapeutic outcomes. Some specific variants like TSC2 and FANCD2 in head and neck cancer can help in analysing patients mainly based on their likelihood of adverse effects. This helps in developing protocols according to the needs of the patient to reduce complications and improve efficacy (Deichaite et al., 2022).

Prognostic Biomarkers in Lung Cancer

NSCLC explains the usage of biomarkers in the clinical decision-making process. Some biomarkers like FN1 and THBS1 were identified as predictors of tumour response to RT. They helped in creating personalized plans for improving tumour control and reducing systemic toxicity (Li et al., 2022). Also circulating tumour DNA (ctDNA) is another emerging biomarker that can help in real-time monitoring of treatment responses and guide in adaptive therapy strategies. The PD-L1 expression also helps in immunotherapy and the determination of RT interactions with the immune system. High levels of PD-L1 can be correlated with better outcomes (Deichaite et al., 2022). Genetic signatures have also become an important biomarker for the prediction of RT outcomes. Analysis among different cancer types has shown a high-predictive accuracy (**Figure 2.5**). The area under the curve (AUC) values range between 0.772 and 0.972. This shows their efficacy in the identification of benefits that patients will receive in RT (Xu et al., 2022).

The selection of immunotherapy or RT in cancer treatment is increasingly guided by specific biomarkers that predict patient response, thereby allowing for more personalized therapeutic approaches. In lung cancer, one of the most well-studied biomarkers is PD-L1 expression. High PD-L1 expression, often defined by thresholds such as ≥1% or ≥50%, is associated with a favourable response to PD-1 inhibitors. This suggests that patients with elevated PD-L1 levels are more likely to benefit from immunotherapy rather than RT (Ntanasis-Stathopoulos et al., 2020). Studies have consistently shown that patients exhibiting high PD-L1 expression experience improved outcomes with agents like pembrolizumab, which has become a cornerstone in the treatment of metastatic NSCLC. The predictive value of PD-L1 not only assists clinicians in selecting the appropriate therapeutic modality but also helps avoid the potential toxicities associated with RT when immunotherapy might offer superior efficacy.

In colorectal cancer, MSI status is a critical biomarker for guiding treatment decisions. Tumours that are classified as MSI-H, often due to defective mismatch repair (dMMR) mechanisms, tend to have a higher mutational burden. This increased mutational load

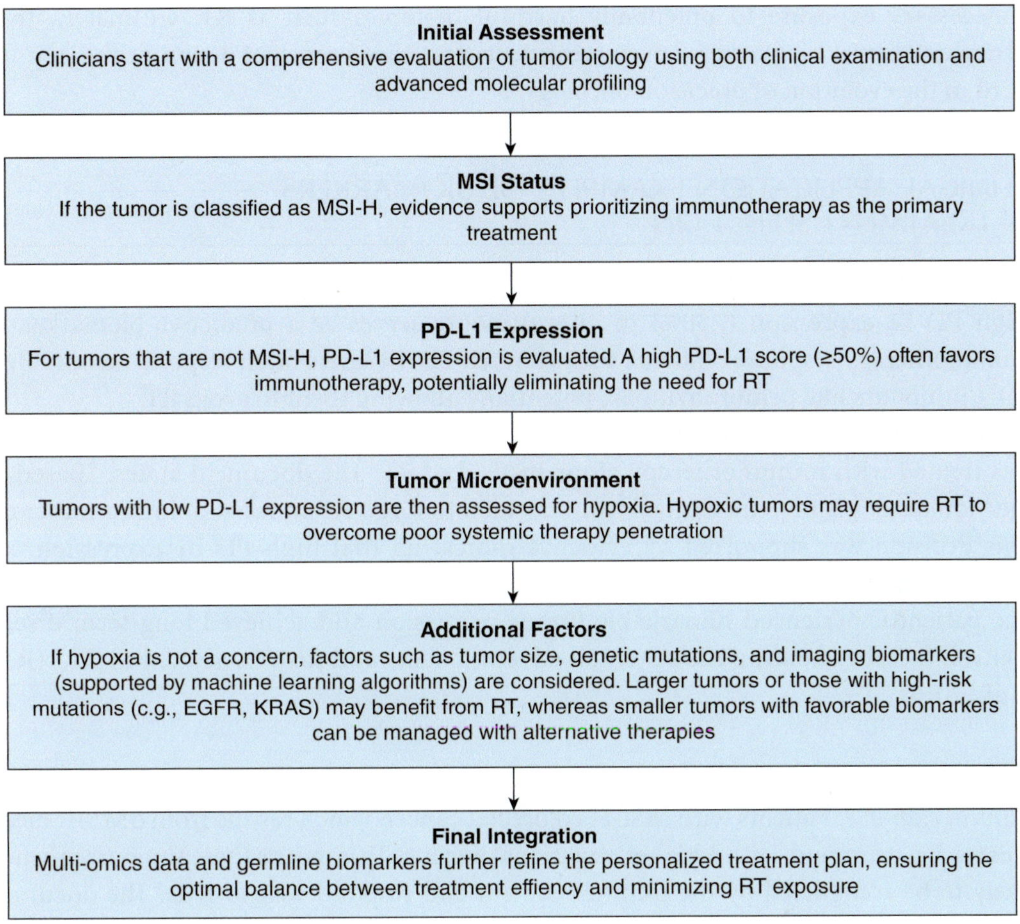

FIGURE 2.5 Decision-making process for selecting treatment strategies based on tumour characteristics.

enhances the likelihood of the tumour being recognized by the immune system, making these tumours more responsive to ICIs. Consequently, patients with MSI-H colorectal cancer often benefit significantly from immunotherapy, which may obviate the need for RT in certain settings (Zang et al., 2019; Chen, 2023).

Conversely, patients with proficient mismatch repair (pMMR) tumours are less likely to respond to immunotherapy, and alternative treatment modalities, including RT, may be more appropriate for achieving local tumour control.

While biomarkers like PD-L1 and MSI provide valuable insights into tumour behaviour and therapeutic response, it is important to note that their predictive power is not absolute. Ongoing research continues to explore additional biomarkers and refine current thresholds to enhance treatment personalization further (Ntanasis-Stathopoulos et al., 2020). Integration of these biomarkers into clinical decision-making supports a more tailored approach, enabling clinicians to maximize treatment efficacy while minimizing unnecessary exposure to potentially harmful therapies such as RT. Ultimately, these advancements in biomarker-driven treatment strategies represent a significant step forward in the evolution of precision oncology.

CLINICAL APPLICATION EXAMPLES OF BIOMARKERS IN TREATMENT SELECTION

PD-L1 Expression in Lung Cancer

High PD-L1 expression (≥50%) in lung tumours serves as a predictive biomarker for immunotherapy response. Patients with elevated PD-L1 levels often respond favourably to PD-1 inhibitors like pembrolizumab, potentially allowing them to avoid RT.

Clinical example: A patient with metastatic NSCLC showing high PD-L1 expression was treated with immunotherapy alone instead of RT. The document states: "Based on the biomarker profile, the clinical team decided to forgo RT in favor of immunotherapy. This decision was supported by evidence indicating that high PD-L1 expression correlates with significant antitumor responses when treated with immunotherapy alone. The patient experienced remarkable tumor regression and achieved long-term disease control, thereby avoiding the potential adverse effects and toxicity related to RT" (Reck et al., 2016).

MSI-H Status in Colorectal Cancer

Clinical example: Patients with MSI-H colorectal cancer, which results from dMMR mechanisms, have tumours with a higher mutational burden. This means these tumours are more likely to be recognized by the immune system and respond well to ICIs. The document states that "patients with MSI-H colorectal cancer often benefit significantly from immunotherapy, which may obviate the need for RT in certain settings" (Le et al., 2017). In contrast, patients with pMMR tumours might still require RTT for effective local control.

Luminal A Breast Cancer

Clinical example: The LUMINA trial focused on women aged 55 years or older with T1N0 luminal A breast cancer. These patients received endocrine therapy without RT, and findings revealed a low 5-year local recurrence rate. This reinforces that RT can be safely omitted in this specific low-risk population based on the molecular subtype.

Hypoxic Tumour Microenvironment

Clinical example: The study describes a patient with a hypoxic lung tumour who required a combination therapy approach: "A patient with a hypoxic lung tumor underwent combination therapy involving radiotherapy (RT) and chemotherapy. Hypoxia, a condition where the tumor experiences low oxygen levels, can lead to treatment resistance, particularly reducing the efficacy of RT when used alone" (Overgaard, 2007). In this case, understanding the TME led clinicians to combine RT with chemotherapy to enhance tumour radiosensitivity and improve drug penetration.

Decipher Genomic Score in Prostate Cancer

Clinical example: The Decipher genomic score helps categorize prostate cancer patients into different risk groups. Patients with low Decipher scores have a reduced likelihood of metastasis and disease progression, allowing them to potentially avoid RT following surgery. The study notes that "by identifying individuals who are at low risk of recurrence, the Decipher score not only minimizes exposure to the potential side effects of RT but also supports a more cost-effective treatment paradigm" (Den et al., 2015).

Oncotype DX in Breast Cancer

Clinical example: The Oncotype DX assay evaluates the expression of 21 genes within breast tumour tissue to generate a recurrence score. For patients with early-stage hormone receptor-positive breast cancer, a low Oncotype DX score suggests minimal benefit from adjuvant therapies. The article states that "these patients might also be considered for a no-radiotherapy approach, particularly if other favorable clinical parameters are present" (Paik et al., 2004).

These examples demonstrate how biomarker-driven treatment decisions are transforming cancer care by enabling more personalized approaches that can safely omit RT in appropriate cases.

TUMOUR BIOLOGY IMPACT ON TREATMENT

Tumour biology plays a pivotal role in tailoring cancer treatment strategies, as demonstrated by real-world case studies that integrate molecular and microenvironmental data to guide clinical decisions. For instance, in lung cancer management, assessing the TME is crucial. In one case study, noted earlier, a patient with a hypoxic lung tumour underwent combination therapy involving RT and chemotherapy. Hypoxia, a condition where the tumour experiences low oxygen levels, can lead to treatment resistance, particularly reducing the efficacy of RT when used alone. Recognizing this, clinicians opted to combine RT with chemotherapy to enhance tumour radiosensitivity and improve drug penetration. This integrated approach successfully overcame the challenges posed by hypoxia, resulting in improved tumour control and better overall survival outcomes (Peng et al., 2023). This case underlines the necessity for a detailed evaluation of the TME to determine the optimal treatment regimen.

In another case, also mentioned earlier, the role of biomarkers in guiding treatment decisions is highlighted by a patient with high PD-L1 expression. Elevated PD-L1 levels in tumours are associated with a favourable response to ICIs, specifically PD-1/PD-L1 inhibitors. Based on the biomarker profile, the clinical team decided to forgo RT in favour of immunotherapy. This decision was supported by evidence indicating that high PD-L1 expression correlates with significant anti-tumour responses when treated with immunotherapy alone. The patient experienced remarkable tumour regression and achieved long-term disease control, thereby avoiding the potential adverse effects and toxicity related to RT (Yang et al., 2022; Smith et al., 2024). This case exemplifies how biomarker-driven treatment pathways can lead to effective, less invasive treatment alternatives.

These examples illustrate the transformative impact of tumour biology on clinical decision- making. By incorporating factors such as hypoxia and PD-L1 expression, clinicians can better predict treatment responses and personalize therapy, thus maximizing efficacy while minimizing unnecessary toxicity. However, it is essential to note that while these biomarkers provide critical insights, they are only one piece of the puzzle. Other factors, including patient comorbidities, genetic predispositions and individual treatment preferences, must also be considered to achieve a truly holistic and effective treatment plan (Peng et al., 2023). Integrating comprehensive biomarker analysis with a patient-centred approach ultimately enhances treatment personalization and advances the practice of precision oncology.

Artificial intelligence (AI) is increasingly becoming a cornerstone in the optimization of cancer treatment, particularly for lung cancer patients. By harnessing advanced algorithms and integrating diverse data types, AI plays a crucial role in selecting patients who may benefit from systemic therapy alone, thereby avoiding unnecessary RT. Tools such as RaySearch and IBM Watson are at the forefront of this revolution, utilizing sophisticated data analytics to process molecular, radiomic and clinical data. This integrated approach not only enhances treatment efficacy but also significantly improves patients' quality of life by reducing exposure to the adverse effects of RT (Ladbury et al., 2023; El Sabrouty & Elouadi, 2024).

AI IN PATIENT SELECTION FOR NO-RT

AI-driven predictive modelling has transformed how clinicians assess patient eligibility for NO-RT. By analysing complex datasets, AI models can forecast which patients are likely to respond well to systemic therapies alone. This approach minimizes the need for RT, sparing patients from its potential toxicities. Predictive algorithms evaluate factors such as tumour histology, molecular profile and radiomic features extracted from imaging studies. For instance, in lung cancer, the integration of clinical, genomic and imaging data allows AI to generate a comprehensive view of a patient's profile, which in turn informs a personalized treatment plan (Pachika et al., 2024; Mishra & Bisht, 2024).

Data integration is critical in this context. AI systems assimilate diverse data streams—including electronic health records, genomic sequencing results and advanced imaging outputs—to produce actionable insights. This integration supports a nuanced understanding of tumour biology and patient-specific variables, enabling clinicians to predict treatment responses with greater accuracy. As a result, patients who are ideal candidates for systemic therapy alone can be identified early, thus avoiding the unnecessary risks associated with RT.

Quality-of-Life Considerations

The impact of AI-driven treatment optimization extends beyond traditional survival metrics. Quality of life is a paramount consideration, especially in cancers like lung cancer, where treatment side effects can severely affect patient wellbeing. For instance, reducing RT exposure can be particularly beneficial for young brain tumour patients by preserving cognitive health and memory function (Tuncel & Cakir, 2024). AI-driven decision-making processes prioritize not only survival but also overall patient wellbeing, aligning treatment regimens with individual health goals and lifestyle considerations (El Sabrouty & Elouadi, 2024).

ADVANCES IN TREATMENT OPTIMIZATION AND ADAPTIVE RADIOTHERAPY

Modern technologies such as adaptive radiotherapy, AI-driven treatment planning and dynamic imaging are pivotal in refining radiation doses and strategies, ultimately improving patient selection for NO-RT (Martin et al., 2016).

The continuous evolution of treatment optimization technologies has led to significant advancements in adaptive RT. Adaptive RT leverages real-time imaging to adjust treatment plans dynamically, accounting for tumour movement and anatomical changes during the treatment course. This approach ensures precise dose delivery to the target while sparing surrounding healthy tissues, thus reducing toxicity risks (Rath et al., 2025). The real-time adaptation afforded by these systems is especially beneficial in lung cancer, where respiratory motion can lead to significant anatomical variations.

AI-driven treatment planning is another area where technology is making a substantial impact. Algorithms can automate complex tasks such as tumour delineation and dose prediction, thereby streamlining the planning process and reducing the time required for treatment preparation. Systems developed by companies such as RaySearch and IBM Watson are capable of automating contouring tasks, optimizing radiation dose distribution and even suggesting modifications based on patient-specific anatomical and biological characteristics (Al Hagawi et al., 2024; Kisia, 2025). These innovations not only enhance treatment precision but also free up valuable time for clinicians to focus on patient care.

Dynamic imaging techniques, such as multimodal imaging, further complement these advances. Functional MRI and PET-CT provide real-time insights into tumour physiology, enabling clinicians to assess the biological response to treatment and adjust doses accordingly (Rath et al., 2025). This dynamic imaging capability is a critical component of modern RT, allowing for a more personalized approach that adapts to changes in tumour behaviour over time.

Technical Innovations: Dose Painting and Multicriteria Optimization

Among the technical innovations in RT, dose painting stands out as a method that allows for differential radiation dose distribution within a tumour. By targeting regions of the tumour that exhibit higher biological activity or resistance, dose painting ensures that these areas receive a higher radiation dose, while sparing normal tissues (Kumar et al., 2025). This method is particularly useful for tumours with heterogeneous characteristics, as it tailors the treatment to the tumour's internal variability.

Multicriteria optimization is another breakthrough that has improved RT planning. This technique incorporates various treatment objectives such as tumour control probability and normal tissue complication probability into the planning process. By balancing these objectives, clinicians can develop treatment plans that maximize therapeutic efficacy while minimizing the risk of adverse effects (Gao et al., 2025). This optimization is crucial in scenarios where trade-offs between different clinical priorities must be carefully managed.

RECENT OPTIMIZATION ADVANCES

Adaptive Radiotherapy

This approach utilizes real-time imaging to adjust treatment plans based on tumour movement and anatomical changes, ensuring precise dose delivery (Rath et al., 2025). Adaptive radiotherapy has demonstrated efficacy in enhancing target accuracy while minimizing exposure to surrounding healthy tissues, reducing toxicity risks.

AI-Driven Treatment Planning

AI algorithms streamline the treatment planning process, significantly reducing planning time and improving accuracy in tumour delineation and dose prediction (Al Hagawi et al., 2024; Kisia, 2025). AI-driven systems can automate contouring tasks and optimize radiation dose distribution, ensuring personalized treatment strategies.

Dynamic Imaging

Techniques such as multimodal imaging enhance tumour tracking and response assessment, allowing for tailored treatment adjustments (Rath et al., 2025). Methods such as functional MRI and PET-CT provide real-time insights into tumour physiology, enabling dose adaptation based on biological response.

TECHNICAL DETAILS

Dose Painting

This method enables differential radiation dose distribution within the tumour, targeting heterogeneous tumour regions with high precision while sparing surrounding normal tissues (Kumar et al., 2025). Dose painting is particularly beneficial for tumours exhibiting high biological variability, ensuring effective treatment.

Multicriteria Optimization

This technique incorporates multiple treatment objectives, optimizing plans based on clinical priorities and patient-specific factors (Gao et al., 2025). By balancing trade-offs such as tumour control probability and normal tissue complication probability, multicriteria optimization enhances decision-making in RT planning.

Real-Time Adaptive Techniques

These methods adjust treatment delivery based on immediate feedback from imaging systems, enhancing tumour control and reducing unnecessary radiation exposure (Kisia, 2025). Real-time adaptation is particularly useful in cases with significant anatomical changes, such as head and neck and lung cancers.

Ongoing research focuses on integrating ML and AI to refine RT planning further. Promising approaches aim to develop interpretable AI systems that enhance personalized care while addressing challenges in clinical workflows (Al Hagawi et al., 2024). AI-driven predictive modelling is being explored to optimize fractionation schemes, predict treatment responses and minimize radiation-induced toxicity. While these advancements present significant opportunities for improving RT, challenges such as data privacy, regulatory approval and the interpretability of AI models remain critical barriers to widespread implementation. Future research should emphasize developing robust AI frameworks that integrate seamlessly into clinical workflows, ensuring both efficacy and safety in radiation therapy decision-making (Wallace et al., 2025).

REAL-TIME ADAPTIVE TECHNIQUES AND FUTURE DIRECTIONS

Real-time adaptive techniques represent the cutting edge of RT planning. These methods continuously adjust the treatment based on immediate feedback from imaging systems, which is particularly valuable for cancers like lung and head and neck cancers, where anatomical changes can be pronounced. Real-time adaptation not only enhances tumour control but also reduces unnecessary radiation exposure, contributing to a better safety profile for patients (Kisia, 2025).

The integration of AI into these processes holds immense promise. AI-driven predictive modelling is being developed to optimize fractionation schemes, predict treatment responses and minimize radiation-induced toxicity. Despite these advances, challenges such as data quality, standardization and regulatory approval persist, and there remains a critical need for ongoing research and collaboration in this field (Mishra & Bisht, 2024).

The combination of AI and advanced RT techniques is revolutionizing the management of lung cancer by enhancing patient selection, optimizing treatment planning and ultimately improving quality of life. Through sophisticated data integration, dynamic imaging and adaptive planning, AI enables a personalized, evidence-based approach that reduces unnecessary exposure to RT and tailors treatment to the unique biological characteristics of each tumour. As AI continues to evolve, its role in radiation oncology will expand, driving further improvements in patient outcomes and heralding a new era of precision oncology (Ladbury et al., 2023; Al Hagawi et al., 2024; El Sabrouty & Elouadi, 2024; Kisia, 2025; Rath et al., 2025).

TUMOUR TYPES

Early-Stage Breast Cancer

Research by Whelan et al. (2023) suggested that patients with luminal A breast cancer may avoid RT after surgery without compromising local control. The LUMINA study has stated that the local recurrence rate is only 2.3% in patients who receive endocrine therapy alone. This highlights the potential to avoid RT in some selected low-risk patients and also reduces the burden of treatment.

Age and Tumour Characteristics

Older patients over 65 years have shown lower local recurrence rates with NO-RT. The PRIME II trial has evaluated the recurrence rate of 4.1% at 5 years in older women treated with breast-conserving surgery alone. This shows the feasibility of avoiding RT in this population (Kunkler et al., 2023). The status of oestrogen receptors also significantly affects the recurrence risk. High oestrogen receptor tumours have a lower likelihood of recurrence when compared to low oestrogen receptor tumours. From this, it can be observed that the status of oestrogen is also crucial in cancer treatment decisions (Wen et al., 2016; Purswani et al., 2022).

Implications for Treatment

It is essential to select patients carefully for NO-RT. Some factors like age, tumour subtype and molecular profiling are important in the identification of low-risk patients. These patients may undergo NO-RT (Purswani et al., 2022). Some studies state that the local recurrence rate may increase slightly without RT; however, the overall survival rate remains comparable. A study (Kunkler et al., 2015) supports NO-RT as an option for the selection of low-risk patients. However, for patients of a young age or those who have high-risk tumour characteristics, the personalized treatment plan remains important for reducing the risks (Dowidar et al., 2024).

Recent Clinical Trial Evidence on NO-RT Approaches

Recent clinical trials have evaluated the omission of RT in select low-risk breast cancer patients, demonstrating promising outcomes in terms of local recurrence, overall survival and quality-of-life endpoints. Trials such as PRIME II, CALGB 9343 and LUMINA provide substantial evidence supporting the safety and efficacy of omitting RT in specific populations (Wang et al., 2021).

KEY TRIALS AND OUTCOMES

PRIME II

The PRIME II trial investigated whether omitting RT in older women with early-stage breast cancer affects clinical outcomes. This study included women aged 65 years or older with T1–2, N0, M0 hormone receptor-positive breast cancer treated with breast-conserving surgery and endocrine therapy. Patients were randomized to receive either RT or NO-RT. The 5-year local recurrence rate was 4.1% in the NO-RT group compared to 1.3% in the RT group, with no significant differences in overall survival (93.8% vs. 94.2%) (Kunkler et al., 2013).

CALGB 9343

CALGB 9343 evaluated RT omission in women aged 70 years or older with early-stage hormone receptor-positive breast cancer. Participants underwent breast-conserving surgery and endocrine therapy, with randomization to RT or NO-RT. The study found that omitting RT did not significantly impact overall survival or local recurrence rates, further supporting the feasibility of an NO-RT approach in select elderly patients (Aebi et al., 2012).

TABLE 2.1 Summary of Key Trial Endpoints

Trial Name	Patient Population	Treatment Arms	Local Recurrence Rate	Overall Survival Rate
PRIME II	Women ≥65, early breast cancer	RT vs. NO-RT	4.1% (NO-RT)	93.8% (NO-RT)
CALGB 9343	Women ≥70, early-stage breast cancer	RT vs. NO-RT	Not specified	Not specified
LUMINA	Women ≥55, T1N0 luminal A breast cancer	NO-RT	Low	Not specified

LUMINA

The LUMINA trial focused on women aged 55 years or older with T1N0 luminal A breast cancer who received endocrine therapy without RT (**Table 2.1**). Findings revealed a low 5-year local recurrence rate, reinforcing that RT can be safely omitted in this specific low-risk population (Whelan et al., 2022).

These findings suggest that in carefully selected low-risk patients, omitting RT can be a safe and effective strategy. However, clinical decision-making should consider individual patient factors, tumour characteristics and long-term implications. Ongoing trials such as IDEA continue to explore RT omission strategies, providing further insights into optimizing treatment for low-risk breast cancer patients.

NON-SURGICAL APPROACHES IN LUNG CANCER

The management of early-stage NSCLC using non-surgical methods has improved in recent years. Some of the techniques used are SBRT and radiofrequency ablation (RFA). These techniques provide efficient control of tumours with minimal invasiveness by making them suitable for patients who are medically inoperable or who try to avoid surgery.

SBRT had shown over 90% of local control rates and 97% of overall survival rates in 2 years. This shows that SBRT provides impressive outcomes for NSCLCs that are inoperable (Kocak Uzel et al., 2023). Peripheral tumours are related to low toxicity profiles, while central tumours may have high risks due to proximity to critical structures such as the heart and major airways (Csiki et al., 2024; Lyu & Wei, 2024). SBRT is recommended for patients who have early-stage NSCLC and cannot undergo surgery because of some comorbidities, age or poor pulmonary reserve (Martin et al., 2023). RFA uses thermal energy to ablate cancer cells and provides a minimally invasive and precise treatment option for localized tumours (Pham, 2023). It was mainly effective in small and peripheral NSCLC tumours. RFA can often be performed on an outpatient basis, helping to improve convenience and reduction of hospital stays (Csiki et al., 2024).

CASE EXAMPLES

RT can be avoided strategically in certain clinical scenarios where tumour biology and its related risks are more than their benefits. This approach ensures that the treatment is to reduce harm and also optimize the outcomes for specific patient populations. Some of the examples are provided next.

TUMOUR-INDUCED METASTASIS RISKS

RT may sometimes inadvertently improve the potential of metastasis by various mechanisms. For example, low-dose ionizing radiation has the effect of promoting angiogenesis. This can help in tumour growth and can also affect the adjacent tissues (Sofia Vala et al., 2010). Also, RT-induced changes in the phenotype of tumour cells, like EMT, may lead to an increase in metastasis and invasiveness (Blyth et al., 2018). In these types of cases, systemic therapies such as chemotherapy or any targeted agents can be used instead of RT to reduce the risks.

NEUROCOGNITIVE CONCERNS IN PAEDIATRIC PATIENTS

In paediatric patients with medulloblastoma, mainly infants may have neurocognitive side effects of craniospinal irradiation (CSI), which means it may be necessary to opt for alternative treatment methods. Studies have reported that chemotherapy-alone protocols can help in improving intellectual outcomes when compared to conventional CSI that reduces long-term neurodevelopmental impairment (Lafay-Cousin et al., 2009). This highlights the significance of preserving the quality of life in young patients and also managing the disease effectively.

AGGRESSIVE TUMOUR BIOLOGY IN BREAST CANCER

For patients who have aggressive breast cancer phenotypes such as triple-negative or HER2-positive tumours, surgical methods such as mastectomy may be used instead of breast-conserving therapy with RT. These decisions are made by considering the high risk of local recurrence rates related to aggressive tumour biology mainly in node-positive disease (Mittendorf & Bedrosian, 2014).

ABSCOPAL EFFECT CONSIDERATIONS

It may be necessary to avoid RT sometimes; however, certain types of tumours show a paradoxical advantage from low-dose RT due to the abscopal effect. This phenomenon involves systemic immune responses triggered by localized RT and potentially improves the outcomes in a metastatic environment (Morita et al., 2022). These immunomodulatory effects demonstrate the role of RT in cancer treatment, balancing its risks and benefits based on tumour biology.

TAKEAWAYS

This chapter emphasizes the critical role of tumour biology in guiding treatment strategies, particularly concerning the decision to utilize or forgo RT. The intricate relationship between tumour characteristics, patient-specific factors and emerging scientific data forms the foundation for personalized treatment approaches that significantly enhance patient outcomes.

Key Factors Influencing Treatment Decisions

- *Tumour Characteristics*: Understanding specific tumour features, such as growth rate, molecular profile, size and potential for metastasis, is paramount in determining appropriate treatment strategies. For instance, tumours with high rates of PD-L1 expression often respond well to immunotherapy, potentially negating the need for RT. Conversely, larger tumours or those exhibiting hypoxia may still benefit from RT to ensure effective local control.

- *Biomarkers and Genetic Profiling*: The use of biomarkers and genetic profiling is essential for predicting tumour responses to RT. These tools help in identifying which patients can safely avoid RT, thus reducing unnecessary radiation exposure. For example, early-stage hormone receptor-positive breast cancer patients may be candidates for a NO-RT approach based on their specific tumour biology and associated risk profiles.
- *TME*: The TME plays a significant role in treatment response. Factors such as hypoxia and the presence of immune-suppressive elements can affect the efficacy of RT. Understanding these interactions allows for the development of strategies that can either enhance the effectiveness of RT or, in some cases, avoid it altogether.
- *Personalized Treatment Plans*: Integrating tumour biology into clinical decision-making fosters a personalized approach to treatment. By considering individual patient factors, such as comorbidities and genetic predispositions, healthcare professionals can tailor treatment plans that maximize efficacy while minimizing adverse effects.

Importance of NO-RT

- *Risk–Benefit Analysis*: The decision to proceed with or omit RT must be made through a thorough risk–benefit analysis. Factors such as local recurrence rates, overall survival rates and potential long-term risks associated with RT must be weighed carefully. For example, the PRIME II and CALGB 9343 trials have shown that selected older patients with low-risk early-stage breast cancer can safely forgo RT without compromising survival outcomes.
- *Clinical Case Studies*: Real-world examples illustrate the successful application of NO-RT protocols. In patients with early-stage low-risk cancers, studies have demonstrated that omitting RT can lead to comparable outcomes in terms of survival and recurrence rates. Such findings reinforce the need for individualized treatment strategies based on tumour biology rather than a one-size-fits-all approach.
- *Technological Innovations*: Advances in treatment technologies, including adaptive radiotherapy and AI-driven planning systems, enhance the ability to refine treatment regimens according to tumour characteristics. These innovations allow for better patient selection for NO-RT by ensuring that only those who would genuinely benefit from RT are exposed to it.
- *Balancing Efficacy and Safety*: The overarching goal of integrating tumour biology into treatment decisions is to achieve a balance between therapeutic efficacy and safety. By understanding the unique biological characteristics of tumours, clinicians can make more informed decisions that ultimately improve the quality of life for patients while effectively managing their cancer.

CONCLUSION

This chapter highlights the significant role of tumour biology in the determination of the appropriateness of RT. This chapter insists on the necessity of balancing risks and benefits for optimal patient outcomes. By understanding the specific characteristics of a tumour, including growth rate, molecular profile and microenvironmental influences, can determine the approach in which the personalized treatment can be designed. The current challenges are tumour heterogeneity, hypoxia and genetic mutations; however, they also provide opportunities for targeted interventions that include tumour environment modulation and employment of molecular-guided therapies. Emerging tools like biomarkers and genetic profiling have revolutionized treatment planning by allowing clinicians to predict RT responses and minimize unnecessary exposure. Real-world examples like NO-RT protocols for early-stage hormone receptor-positive breast cancer and well-differentiated thyroid cancers state the potential for personalized and patient-centred care. These cases show how these advancements in tumour biology can effectively help patients by optimizing therapeutic efficacy while reducing adverse effects.

Furthermore, the chapter discusses technological innovations and the integration of ML frameworks in identifying predictive biomarkers. These advancements refine RT protocols by aligning them with individual tumour profiles. By exploring risk versus benefit analyses, the importance of precise decision-making in tailoring RT to specific cancer types and patient needs is observed. In conclusion, understanding tumour biology not only advances oncologic care but also paves the way for more refined and patient-specific therapies. This foundational knowledge helps in shifting towards evidence-based approaches by improving the treatment efficacy and quality of life for cancer patients.

REFERENCES

Aebi, S., Gelber, S., Láng, I., Anderson, S., Robidoux, A., Martín, M., Nortier, J., Mamounas, E., Geyer, C., Maibach, R., Gelber, R., Wolmark, N., & Wapnir, I. (2012). Abstract S3-2: Chemotherapy prolongs survival for isolated local or regional recurrence of breast cancer: The CALOR trial (Chemotherapy as Adjuvant for Locally Recurrent breast cancer; IBCSG 27-02, NSABP B-37, BIG 1-02). *Cancer Research*, *72*(24_Supplement), S3-2–S3-2. https://doi.org/10.1158/0008-5472.SABCS12-S3-2

Al Hagawi, W. S. A., Jubran, E. A. H., Almohammedsaleh, F. Y. A., Ayed, A. S., Hamdi, A. N. A., Alnasser, A. M., Alosaimy, O. M., Alshammari, T. A., Alghamdi, A. H. J., Alghamdi, A. M. J., Al Shammari, T. F., Maqadi, A. A. A., Almutairi, F. K. M., & Alhusainiah, H. H. H. (2024). Integrating artificial intelligence in radiotherapy: Challenges and opportunities in clinical workflows. *Journal of Ecohumanism*, *3*(8). https://doi.org/10.62754/joe.v3i8.5552

Ancel, J., Perotin, J.-M., Dewolf, M., Launois, C., Mulette, P., Nawrocki-Raby, B., Dalstein, V., Gilles, C., Deslée, G., Polette, M., & Dormoy, V. (2021). Hypoxia in lung cancer management: A translational approach. *Cancers*, *13*(14), 3421. https://doi.org/10.3390/cancers13143421

Andersson, B., Langen, B., Liu, P., & Dávila López, M. (2023). Development of a machine learning framework for radiation biomarker discovery and absorbed dose prediction. *Frontiers in Oncology*, *13*, 1156009. https://doi.org/10.3389/fonc.2023.1156009

Barsoumian, H. B., Sheth, R. A., Ramapriyan, R., Hsu, E., Gagea, M., Crowley, K., Sezen, D., Williams, M., & Welsh, J. W. (2023). Radiation therapy modulates tumor physical characteristics to reduce intratumoral pressure and enhance intratumoral drug delivery and retention. *Advances in Radiation Oncology*, *8*(2), 101137. https://doi.org/10.1016/j.adro.2022.101137

Bennett, B. (2021). A closure look on benefits of radiation therapy. *Journal of Cancer Science & Therapy*, *12*, 428.

Blecharz, P., Reinfuss, M., Jakubowicz, J., Skotnicki, P., Łuczyńska, E., Bodzek, M., & Urbański, K. (2013). Radiation therapy complications in patients with primary invasive vaginal carcinoma. *Polish Gynaecology*, *84*(3). https://doi.org/10.17772/gp/1564

Blyth, B. J., Cole, A. J., MacManus, M. P., & Martin, O. A. (2018). Radiation therapy-induced metastasis: Radiobiology and clinical implications. *Clinical & Experimental Metastasis, 35*(4), 223–236. https://doi.org/10.1007/s10585-017-9867-5

Chen, K. (2023). Biomarkers and immunotherapy for colorectal cancer. *Highlights in Science, Engineering and Technology, 36*, 1356–1366. https://doi.org/10.54097/hset.v36i.6252

Chen, Y., Dai, X., Wang, J., Tao, C., Wang, Y., Zhu, Q., Wang, Z., Zhang, T., Lan, Q., & Zhao, J. (2023). Heterogenous profiles between primary lung cancers and paired brain metastases reveal tumor evolution. *Frontiers in Oncology, 13*, 1026099. https://doi.org/10.3389/fonc.2023.1026099

Cheng, S. H., Jian, J. J.-M., Chan, K.-Y., Tsai, S. Y. C., Liu, M.-C., & Chen, C.-M. (1998). The benefit and risk of postmastectomy radiation therapy in patients with high-risk breast cancer. *American Journal of Clinical Oncology, 21*(1), 12–17. https://doi.org/10.1097/00000421-199802000-00003

Chorbińska, J., Krajewski, W., & Zdrojowy, R (2021). Urological complications after radiation therapy—Nothing ventured, nothing gained: A narrative review. *Translational Cancer Research, 10*(2), 1096–1118. https://doi.org/10.21037/tcr-20-2589

Cooper, G. M. (2000). The development and causes of cancer. In *The Cell: A Molecular Approach*. 2nd Edition. Sinauer Associates. https://www.ncbi.nlm.nih.gov/books/NBK9963/

Csiki, E., Simon, M., Papp, J., Barabás, M., Mikáczó, J., Gál, K., Sipos, D., & Kovács, Á. (2024). Stereotactic body radiotherapy in lung cancer: A contemporary review. *Pathology and Oncology Research, 30*, 1611709. https://doi.org/10.3389/pore.2024.1611709

Dalfovo, D., Scandino, R., Paoli, M., Valentini, S., & Romanel, A. (2024). Germline determinants of aberrant signaling pathways in cancer. *NPJ Precision Oncology, 8*(1), 57. https://doi.org/10.1038/s41698-024-00546-5

Deichaite, I., Hopper, A., Krockenberger, L., Sears, T. J., Sutton, L., Ray, X., Sharabi, A., Navon, A., Sanghvi, P., Carter, H., & Moiseenko, V. (2022). Germline genetic biomarkers to stratify patients for personalized radiation treatment. *Journal of Translational Medicine, 20*(1), 360. https://doi.org/10.1186/s12967-022-03561-x

Den, R. B., Feng, F. Y., Showalter, T. N., et al. (2015). Genomic prostate cancer classifier predicts biochemical failure and metastases in patients after postoperative radiation therapy. *International Journal of Radiation Oncology, Biology, Physics, 91*(3), 555–565.

Dhruba, S. R., Sahni, S., Wang, B., Wu, D., Rajagopal, P. S., Schmidt, Y., Shulman, E. D., Sinha, S., Sammut, S.-J., Caldas, C., Wang, K., & Ruppin, E. (2024). The expression patterns of different cell types and their interactions in the tumor microenvironment are predictive of breast cancer patient response to neoadjuvant chemotherapy. *bioRxiv*. https://doi.org/10.1101/2024.06.14.598770

Dowidar, A., Abdeltwab, Z., Semary, S., & Mohamed, S. (2024). Difference in outcome between luminal a, luminal b in early stage breast cancer retrospective study. *Egyptian Journal of Medical Research, 5*(2), 61–81. https://doi.org/10.21608/ejmr.2023.174543.1293

El Sabrouty, R., & Elouadi, A. (2024). Harnessing AI for precision oncology: Transformative advances in non-small cell lung cancer treatment. *Statistics, Optimization & Information Computing, 13*(1), 347–367. https://doi.org/10.19139/soic-2310-5070-2078

Erdmann-Pham, D. D., Batra, S. S., Turkalo, T. K., Durbin, J., Blanchette, M., Yeh, I., Shain, H., Bastian, B. C., Song, Y. S., Rokhsar, D. S., & Hockemeyer, D. (2023). Tracing cancer evolution and heterogeneity using Hi-C. *Nature Communications, 14*(1), 7111. https://doi.org/10.1038/s41467-023-42651-2

Ferguson, L. R., Chen, H., Collins, A. R., Connell, M., Damia, G., Dasgupta, S., Malhotra, M., Meeker, A. K., Amedei, A., Amin, A., Ashraf, S. S., Aquilano, K., Azmi, S., Bhakta, D., Bilsland, A., Boosani, C. S., Chen, S., Ciriolo, M. R., Fujii, H., … Maxwell, C. A. (2015). Genomic instability in human cancer: Molecular insights and opportunities for therapeutic attack and prevention through diet and nutrition. *Seminars in Cancer Biology, 35*(Suppl), S5. https://doi.org/10.1016/j.semcancer.2015.03.005

Gao, R., Diallo, M., Liu, H., Magliari, A., Sackett, J., Verbakel, W., Meyers, S., Zarepisheh, M., Mcbeth, R., Arberet, S., Kraus, M., Ghesu, F. C., & Kamen, A. (2025). Automating high quality RT planning at scale. *arXiv*. https://doi.org/10.48550/ARXIV.2501.11803

Glaviano, A., Foo, A. S. C., Lam, H. Y., Yap, K. C. H., Jacot, W., Jones, R. H., Eng, H., Nair, M. G., Makvandi, P., Geoerger, B., Kulke, M. H., Baird, R. D., Prabhu, J. S., Carbone, D., Pecoraro, C., Teh, D. B. L., Sethi, G., Cavalieri, V., Lin, K. H., … Kumar, P. (2023). PI3K/AKT/mTOR signaling transduction pathway and targeted therapies in cancer. *Molecular Cancer*, *22*(1), 138. https://doi.org/10.1186/s12943-023-01827-6

Goenka, A., Khan, F., Verma, B., Sinha, P., Dmello, C. C., Jogalekar, M. P., Gangadaran, P., & Ahn, B. (2023). Tumor microenvironment signaling and therapeutics in cancer progression. *Cancer Communications*, *43*(5), 525–561. https://doi.org/10.1002/cac2.12416

Han, X., Burrows, M., Kim, L. C., Xu, J. P., Vostrejs, W., Van Le, T. N., Poltorack, C., Jiang, Y., Cukierman, E., Stanger, B. Z., Reiss, K. A., Shaffer, S. M., Mesaros, C., Keith, B., & Simon, M. C. (2024). Cancer-associated fibroblasts maintain critical pancreatic cancer cell lipid homeostasis in the tumor microenvironment. *Cell Reports*, *43*(11), 114972. https://doi.org/10.1016/j.celrep.2024.114972

He, Y., Sun, M. M., Zhang, G. G., Yang, J., Chen, K. S., Xu, W. W., & Li, B. (2021). Targeting PI3K/Akt signal transduction for cancer therapy. *Signal Transduction and Targeted Therapy*, *6*(1), 425. https://doi.org/10.1038/s41392-021-00828-5

Herlemann, A., Huang, H. -C., Alam, R., Tosoian, J. J., Kim, H. L., Choeurng, V., Sundi, D., Pavlovich, C. P., Han, M., Schaeffer, E. M., Klein, E. A., Lotan, T. L., Ross, A. E., Den, R. B., & Klein, E. A. (2019). Decipher identifies men with otherwise clinically favorable-intermediate risk disease who may not be good candidates for active surveillance. *Prostate Cancer and Prostatic Diseases*, *22*(3), 399–405. https://doi.org/10.1038/s41391-019-0167-9

Jia, S., Bode, A. M., Chen, X., & Luo, X. (2024). Unlocking the potential: Targeting metabolic pathways in the tumor microenvironment for cancer therapy. *Biochimica et Biophysica Acta (BBA) - Reviews on Cancer*, *1879*(5), 189166. https://doi.org/10.1016/j.bbcan.2024.189166

Kim, M., Lee, N. K., Wang, C.-P. J., Lim, J., Byun, M. J., Kim, T.-H., Park, W., Park, D.-H., Kim, S.-N., & Park, C. G. (2023). Reprogramming the tumor microenvironment with biotechnology. *Biomaterials Research*, *27*(1), 5. https://doi.org/10.1186/s40824-023-00343-4

Kisia, N. (2025). Abstract A007: Artificial intelligence in radiation therapy: Bringing in a new era of cancer therapy, accurate and fast. *Clinical Cancer Research*, *31*(2_Supplement), A007. https://doi.org/10.1158/1557-3265.TARGETEDTHERAP-A007

Kleinberg, L. (2010). Does postoperative radiation therapy benefit patients with esophageal cancer? *Journal of Gastrointestinal Oncology*, *1*(2), 70. https://doi.org/10.3978/j.issn.2078-6891.2010.015

Kocak Uzel, E., Bagci Kilic, M., Morcali, H., & Uzel, O. (2023). Stereotactic body radiation therapy for stage I medically operable non-small cell lung cancer. *Scientific Reports*, *13*(1), 10384. https://doi.org/10.1038/s41598-023-37643-7

Kretschmer, A., & Tilki, D. (2017). Biomarkers in prostate cancer—Current clinical utility and future perspectives. *Critical Reviews in Oncology/Hematology*, *120*, 180–193. https://doi.org/10.1016/j.critrevonc.2017.11.004

Kumar, R., Kumar, S., & Singh, Y. P. (2025). Advances in radiation therapy: A comprehensive review of techniques and clinical applications in cancer treatment. *International Journal of Scientific Research in Engineering and Management*, *09*(01), 1–9. https://doi.org/10.55041/IJSREM40477

Kunkler, I., Williams, L., Jack, W., Canney, P., Prescott, R., & Dixon, M. (2013). Abstract S2-01: The PRIME II trial: Wide local excision and adjuvant hormonal therapy ± postoperative whole breast irradiation in women ≥ 65 years with early breast cancer managed by breast conservation. *Cancer Research*, *73*(24_Supplement), S2-01–S2-01. https://doi.org/10.1158/0008-5472.SABCS13-S2-01

Kunkler, I. H., Williams, L. J., Jack, W. J., & Cameron, D. A. (2015). Breast-conserving surgery with or without irradiation in women aged 65 years or older with early breast cancer: A randomised controlled trial. *Lancet Oncology*, *16*(2), 154–163. https://doi.org/10.1016/S1470-2045(14)71221-5

Kunkler, I. H., Williams, L. J., Jack, W. J. L., Cameron, D. A., & Dixon, J. M. (2023). Breast-conserving surgery with or without irradiation in early breast cancer. *New England Journal of Medicine, 388*(7), 585–594. https://doi.org/10.1056/NEJMoa2207586

Ladbury, C., Amini, A., Govindarajan, A., Mambetsariev, I., Raz, D. J., Massarelli, E., Williams, T., Rodin, A., & Salgia, R. (2023). Integration of artificial intelligence in lung cancer: Rise of the machine. *Cell Reports Medicine, 4*(2), 100933. https://doi.org/10.1016/j.xcrm.2023.100933

Lafay-Cousin, L., Bouffet, E., Hawkins, C., Amid, A., Huang, A., & Mabbott, D. J. (2009). Impact of radiation avoidance on survival and neurocognitive outcome in infant medulloblastoma. *Current Oncology, 16*(6), 21–28. https://doi.org/10.3747/co.v16i6.435

LaRiviere, M. J., & Vapiwala, N. (2024). Radiation therapy. In *Penn Clinical Manual of Urology* (pp. 704–734.e5). Elsevier. https://doi.org/10.1016/B978-0-323-77575-5.00028-9

Le, D. T., Durham, J. N., Smith, K. N Wang, H., Bartlett, B. R., Aulakh, L. K., Lu, S., Kemberling, H., Wilt, C., Luber, B. S., Wong, F., Azad, N. S., Rucki, A. A., Laheru, D., Donehower, R., Zaheer, A., Fisher, G. A., Crocenzi, T. S., Lee, J. J., Greten, T. F., … Diaz, L. A., Jr (2017). Mismatch repair deficiency predicts response of solid tumors to PD-1 blockade. *Science, 357*(6349), 409–413. https://doi.org/10.1126/science.aan6733

Li, K., Wang, S., Li, N., Zhao, W., He, N., Wang, J., Ji, K., Zhang, M., Song, H., Liu, Q., & Du, L. (2022). Prognostic biomarkers after radiotherapy for nonsmall cell lung cancer based on bioinformatics analysis. *BioMed Research International, 2022*(1), 9. https://doi.org/10.1155/2022/6405228

Li, L., Zhang, F., Liu, Z., & Fan, Z. (2023). Immunotherapy for triple-negative breast cancer: Combination strategies to improve outcome. *Cancers, 15*(1), 321. https://doi.org/10.3390/cancers15010321

Lyu, Z., & Wei, C. (2024). Stereotactic body radiation therapy (SBRT) for non-small cell lung cancer (NCSLC) therapy. *Cancer Research Journal, 12*(2), 27–35. https://doi.org/10.11648/j.crj.20241202.12

Magill, S. T., Vasudevan, H. N., Seo, K., Villanueva-Meyer, J. E., Choudhury, A., John Liu, S., Pekmezci, M., Findakly, S., Hilz, S., Lastella, S., Demaree, B., Braunstein, S. E., Bush, N. A. O., Aghi, M. K., Theodosopoulos, P. V., Sneed, P. K., Abate, A. R., Berger, M. S., McDermott, M. W., … Raleigh, D. R. (2020). Multiplatform genomic profiling and magnetic resonance imaging identify mechanisms underlying intratumor heterogeneity in meningioma. *Nature Communications, 11*(1), 4803. https://doi.org/10.1038/s41467 020 18582 7

Martin, É., Nicolet, C., Boisselier, P., Khalifa, J., & Thureau, S. (2023). Place de la radiothérapie stéréotaxique pour les cancers bronchiques non à petites cellules de stade I opérables. *Cancer/Radiothérapie, 27*(6–7), 648–652. https://doi.org/10.1016/j.canrad.2023.07.012

Martin, M., Wei, H., & Lu, T. (2016). Targeting microenvironment in cancer therapeutics. *Oncotarget, 7*(32), 52575–52583. https://doi.org/10.18632/oncotarget.9824

Mathema, V. B., Sen, P., Lamichhane, S., Orešič, M., & Khoomrung, S. (2023). Deep learning facilitates multi-data type analysis and predictive biomarker discovery in cancer precision medicine. *Computational and Structural Biotechnology Journal, 21*, 1372–1382. https://doi.org/10.1016/j.csbj.2023.01.043

Mishra, V., & Bisht, S. (2024). The transformative role of ai in radiation oncology. In Loc Nguyen, H S Prashanth, J. Rani Rabha, K. S T S Karthik, C. Raja M, Balaji S R, K. Kumar Jha, C. Sridhar, P. Dutta, Bhavya, M. Solanki, G. N. Vivekananda, M. S. Hossain, R. Roy, B. Sharan, R. Athiakshmi, K. G. Gupta, B. Krishna, … A. Hussain (Eds.), *Futuristic Trends in Artificial Intelligence Volume 3 Book 5* (First, pp. 113–117). Iterative International Publisher, Selfypage Developers Pvt Ltd. https://doi.org/10.58532/V3BBAI5P2CH1

Mittendorf, E. A., & Bedrosian, I. (2014). Breast cancer biology: Implications for local- regional therapy. *Annals of Surgical Oncology, 21*(9), 2820–2822. https://doi.org/10.1245/s10434-014-3730-6

Moores, B. M. (2016). Cost–risk–benefit analysis in diagnostic radiology: A theoretical and economic basis for radiation protection of the patient. *Radiation Protection Dosimetry, 169*(1–4), 2–10. https://doi.org/10.1093/rpd/ncv506

Moran, J. A., Adams, D. L., Edelman, M. J., Lopez, P., He, J., Qiao, Y., Xu, T., Liao, Z., Gardner, K. P., Tang, C.-M., & Lin, S. H. (2022). Monitoring pd-l1 expression on circulating tumor-associated cells in recurrent metastatic non–small-cell lung carcinoma predicts response to immunotherapy with radiation therapy. *JCO Precision Oncology, 6*, e2200457. https://doi.org/10.1200/PO.22.00457

Morita, Y., Saijo, A., Nokihara, H., Mitsuhashi, A., Yoneda, H., Otsuka, K., Ogino, H., Bando, Y., & Nishioka, Y. (2022). Radiation therapy induces an abscopal effect and upregulates programmed death-ligand 1 expression in a patient with non-small cell lung cancer. *Thoracic Cancer, 13*(7), 1079–1082. https://doi.org/10.1111/1759-7714.14330

Ntanasis-Stathopoulos, I., Kyriazoglou, A., Dimopoulos, M. A., & Gavriatopoulou, M. (2020). Clinical biomarkers directing the management of patients with colon and lung cancer (beyond oncogene-addicted NSCLC). *Forum of Clinical Oncology, 11*(1), 3–6. https://doi.org/10.2478/fco-2019-0014

Overgaard, J. (2007). Hypoxic modification of radiotherapy in squamous cell carcinoma of the head and neck—A systematic review and meta-analysis. *Radiotherapy and Oncology, 83*(2), 123–131.

Pachika, P., Valasapalli, S., Ngo, P., & Kloecker, G. (2024). The use of artificial intelligence in lung cancer management. *AI in Precision Oncology, 1*(1), 33–42. https://doi.org/10.1089/aipo.2023.0002

Paik, S., Shak, S., Tang, G., Kim, C., Baker, J., Cronin, M., Baehner, F. L., Walker, M. G., Watson, D., Park, T., Hiller, W., Fisher, E. R., Wickerham, D. L., Bryant, J., & Wolmark, N. (2004). A multigene assay to predict recurrence of tamoxifen-treated, node-negative breast cancer. *New England Journal of Medicine, 351*(27), 2817–2826.

Peng, J., Zhang, L., Wang, L., Feng, H., Yao, D., Meng, R., Liu, X., Li, X., Liu, N., Tan, B., Huang, Z., Li, S., & Meng, X. (2023). Pd-l1 inhibitors combined with thoracic radiotherapy in first-line treatment of extensive stage small cell lung cancer: A propensity score-matched, real-world study. *International Journal of Radiation Oncology*Biology*Physics, 117*(2), S127–S128. https://doi.org/10.1016/j.ijrobp.2023.06.472

Petrucelli, N., Daly, M. B., & Pal, T. (1993). BRCA1- and BRCA2-associated hereditary breast and ovarian cancer. In M. P. Adam, J. Feldman, G. M. Mirzaa, R. A. Pagon, S. E. Wallace & A. Amemiya (Eds.), *GeneReviews*. University of Washington, Seattle. http://www.ncbi.nlm.nih.gov/books/NBK1247/

Pham, L. V. (2023). Ep07. 01-23 stereotactic body radiation therapy for patients with early-stage non-small cell lung cancer inoperable. *Journal of Thoracic Oncology, 18*(11), S518. https://doi.org/10.1016/j.jtho.2023.09.969

Purswani, J. M., Hardy-Abeloos, C., Perez, C. A., Kwa, M. J., Chadha, M., & Gerber, N. K. (2022). Radiation in early-stage breast cancer: Moving beyond an all or nothing approach. *Current Oncology, 30*(1), 184–195. https://doi.org/10.3390/curroncol30010015

Rath, G. K., Devnani, B., Gupta, A. K., & Aggarwal, D. (2025). Technological advances in radiation oncology. *Sarvodaya International Journal of Medicine, 1*(1), 12–14. https://doi.org/10.4103/SIJM.SIJM_3_24

Reck, M., Rodríguez-Abreu, D., Robinson, A. G., Hui, R., Csőszi, T., Fülöp, A., Gottfried, M., Peled, N., Tafreshi, A., Cuffe, S., O'Brien, M., Rao, S., Hotta, K., Leiby, M. A., Lubiniecki, G. M., Shentu, Y., Rangwala, R., Brahmer, J. R., & KEYNOTE-024 Investigators (2016). Pembrolizumab versus chemotherapy for PD-L1–positive non-small-cell lung cancer. *New England Journal of Medicine, 375*(19), 1823–1833.

Smith, G. L. (2016). Toward minimizing overtreatment and undertreatment of ductal carcinoma in situ in the United States. *Journal of Clinical Oncology, 34*(11), 1172–1174. https://doi.org/10.1200/JCO.2015.66.2064

Smith, S., Kao, S., Boyer, M., Franco, M., & Moore, M. (2024). Treatment selection and real-world analysis of immunotherapy with or without chemotherapy in PD-L1-high metastatic non-small cell lung cancer. *Internal Medicine Journal, 54*(8), 1337–1343. https://doi.org/10.1111/imj.16389

Sofia Vala, I., Martins, L. R., Imaizumi, N., Nunes, R. J., Rino, J., Kuonen, F., Carvalho, L. M., Rüegg, C., Grillo, I. M., Barata, J. T., Mareel, M., & Santos, S. C. R. (2010). Low doses of ionizing radiation promote tumor growth and metastasis by enhancing angiogenesis. *PLoS One, 5*(6), e11222. https://doi.org/10.1371/journal.pone.0011222

Sroussi, H. Y., Epstein, J. B., Bensadoun, R., Saunders, D. P., Lalla, R. V., Migliorati, C. A., Heaivilin, N., & Zumsteg, Z. S. (2017). Common oral complications of head and neck cancer radiation therapy: Mucositis, infections, saliva change, fibrosis, sensory dysfunctions, dental caries, periodontal disease, and osteoradionecrosis. *Cancer Medicine, 6*(12), 2918–2931. https://doi.org/10.1002/cam4.1221

Sutera, P., Deek, M. P., Van der Eecken, K., Wyatt, A. W., Kishan, A. U., Molitoris, J. K., Ferris, M. J., Siddiqui, M. M., Rana, Z., Mishra, M. V., Kwok, Y., Davicioni, E., Spratt, D. E., Ost, P., Feng, F. Y., & Tran, P. T. (2022). Genomic biomarkers to guide precision radiotherapy in prostate cancer. *Prostate, 82*(Suppl 1), S73–S85. https://doi.org/10.1002/pros.24373

Tumor Microenvironment. (n.d.). PromoCell. Retrieved February 2, 2025, from https://promocell.com/research-areas/applications-for-our-cancer-media-toolbox/tumor-microenvironment/

Tuncel, N., & Cakir, T. (2024). The role of artificial intelligence (AI) in radiation treatment and investment perspectives. In T. Cakir & N. Tuncel (Eds.), *The Latest Innovative Approaches in Radiation Therapy* (1st ed., pp. 177–220). Nobel Tip Kitabevleri. https://doi.org/10.69860/nobel.9786053359425.8

Valentini, A. M., Cavalcanti, E., Di Maggio, M., & Caruso, M. L. (2018). Ras-expanded mutations and her2 expression in metastatic colorectal cancer: A new step of precision medicine. *Applied Immunohistochemistry & Molecular Morphology, 26*(8), 539–544. https://doi.org/10.1097/PAI.0000000000000475

Vatsyayan, A., & Scaria, V. (2023). Understanding the prevalence of germline oncogenic biomarker variants across the Indian population. https://doi.org/10.1101/2023.10.20.23297298

Wallace, E., & Amemiya, A. (Eds.) (2025). *GeneReviews.* University of Washington, Seattle. http://www.ncbi.nlm.nih.gov/books/NBK1247/

Wang, B., Zhao, Q., Zhang, Y., Liu, Z., Zheng, Z., Liu, S., Meng, L., Xin, Y., & Jiang, X. (2021). Targeting hypoxia in the tumor microenvironment: A potential strategy to improve cancer immunotherapy. *Journal of Experimental & Clinical Cancer Research, 40*(1), 24. https://doi.org/10.1186/s13046-020-01820-7

Wang, Q., Shao, X., Zhang, Y., Zhu, M., Wang, F. X. C., Mu, J., Li, J., Yao, H., & Chen, K. (2023). Role of tumor microenvironment in cancer progression and therapeutic strategy. *Cancer Medicine, 12*(10), 11149–11165. https://doi.org/10.1002/cam4.5698

Wen, G., Zhang, J.-S., Zhang, Y.-J., Zhu, Y.-J., Huang, X.-B., & Guan, X.-X. (2016). Predictive value of molecular subtyping for locoregional recurrence in early-stage breast cancer with n1 without postmastectomy radiotherapy. *Journal of Breast Cancer, 19*(2), 176. https://doi.org/10.4048/jbc.2016.19.2.176

Whelan, T. J., Smith, S., Nielsen, T. O., Parpia, S., Fyles, A. W., Bane, A., Liu, F.-F., Grimard, L., Stevens, C., Bowen, J., Provencher, S., Rakovitch, E., Theberge, V., Mulligan, A. M., Akra, M. A., Voduc, K. D., Hijal, T., Dayes, I. S., Pond, G. R., & Levine, M. N. (2022). LUMINA: A prospective trial omitting radiotherapy (RT) following breast conserving surgery (BCS) in $T_1 N_0$ luminal A breast cancer (BC). *Journal of Clinical Oncology, 40*(17_suppl), LBA501–LBA501. https://doi.org/10.1200/JCO.2022.40.17_suppl.LBA501

Whelan, T. J., Smith, S., Parpia, S., Fyles, A. W., Bane, A., Liu, F.-F., Rakovitch, E., Chang, L., Stevens, C., Bowen, J., Provencher, S., Théberge, V., Mulligan, A. M., Kos, Z., Akra, M. A., Voduc, K. D., Hijal, T., Dayes, I. S., Pond, G., … Levine, M. N. (2023). Omitting radiotherapy after breast-conserving surgery in luminal breast cancer. *New England Journal of Medicine, 389*(7), 612–619. https://doi.org/10.1056/NEJMoa2302344

William, C., Wangmo, C., & Ranjan, A. (2023). Unravelling the application of machine learning in cancer biomarker discovery. *Cancer Insight, 15.* https://doi.org/10.58567/ci02010001

Xiang, M., Chang, D. T., & Pollom, E. L. (2020). Second cancer risk after primary cancer treatment with three-dimensional conformal, intensity-modulated, or proton beam radiation therapy. *Cancer, 126*(15), 3560–3568. https://doi.org/10.1002/cncr.32938

Xiao, S., Klein, L., Petersen, J., Vollmuth, P., Jaeger, P. F., & Maier-Hein, K. H. (2024). Enhancing predictive imaging biomarker discovery through treatment effect analysis. *arXiv*. https://doi.org/10.48550/ARXIV.2406.02534

Xu, Y., Tang, C., Wu, Y., Luo, L., Wang, Y., Wu, Y., & Shi, X. (2022). Prediction of response to radiotherapy by characterizing the transcriptomic features in clinical tumor samples across 15 cancer types. *Computational Intelligence and Neuroscience, 2022*, 1–16. https://doi.org/10.1155/2022/5443709

Yang, R., Wang, D., Li, X., Mao, K., Wang, J., Li, P., Shi, X., Zhang, S., & Wang, Y. (2022). An advanced non-small cell lung cancer patient with EGFR and KRAS mutations, and PD-L1 positive, benefited from immunotherapy: A case report. *Annals of Translational Medicine, 10*(6), 381–381. https://doi.org/10.21037/atm-22-403

Zang, Y., Dai, C., Xu, X., Cai, X., Wang, G., Wei, J., Wu, A., Sun, W., Jiao, S., & Xu, Q. (2019). Comprehensive analysis of potential immunotherapy genomic biomarkers in 1000 Chinese patients with cancer. *Cancer Medicine, 8*(10), 4699–4708. https://doi.org/10.1002/cam4.2381

Zhang, S., Xiao, X., Yi, Y., Wang, X., Zhu, L., Shen, Y., Lin, D., & Wu, C. (2024). Tumor initiation and early tumorigenesis: Molecular mechanisms and interventional targets. *Signal Transduction and Targeted Therapy, 9*(1), 149. https://doi.org/10.1038/s41392-024-01848-7

Surgical Aspects

Examining Surgery's Significance in Tumour Management

Nagesh Madnoorkar and Shantanu Pawar

INTRODUCTION

Surgery plays a significant role in management of tumours and can act as an alternative to radiation therapy (RT) in terms of no radiation therapy (NO-RT) approaches. With advancements in surgical techniques like minimally invasive and organ-sparing surgeries, the surgery can effectively eliminate tumours and also reduce the side effects associated with RT. This chapter evaluates the significance of surgical interventions in cancer treatment and highlights their potential to replace traditional RT methods.

The timeline of surgical advancements over the years, which has facilitated the adoption of the NO-RT approach, is illustrated in **Figure 3.1**.

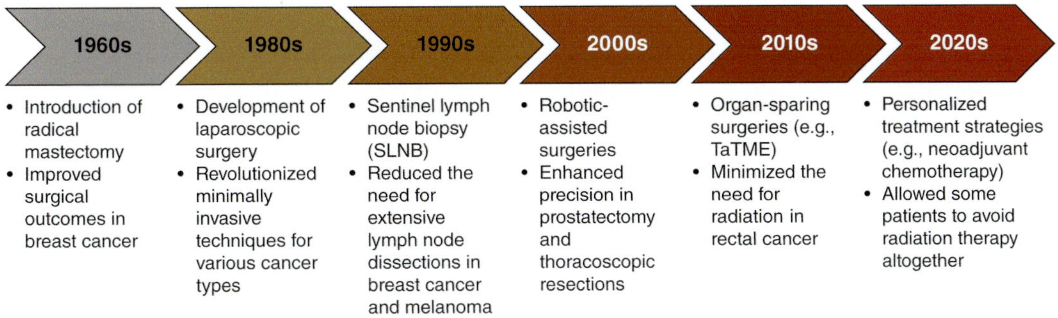

FIGURE 3.1 Timeline of surgical advancements enabling NO-RT.

DOI: 10.1201/9781003529071-3

WHY SURGERY IS CONSIDERED AN ALTERNATIVE TO RADIATION THERAPY

Surgical resection is one of the primary methods used for obtaining complete tumour removal. It provides curative outcomes that can reduce the necessity for adjunct RT in certain malignancies. Advances in surgical oncology like precision resection guided by intraoperative imaging helps in higher rates of margin-negative excision and thus reducing the recurrence risk (Wilson, 1984). In tumours like early-stage breast cancer and head and neck carcinomas, using surgery alone can achieve local control comparable to RT without its associated toxicities (Bibas et al., 2022).

Organ Preservation

By adopting the minimally invasive and robotic-assisted surgeries, the oncological resection was transformed because of more precise tumour excision and preservation of surrounding healthy tissue. Techniques like video-assisted thoracoscopic surgery (VATS) for lung cancer and transanal total mesorectal excision (TaTME) for rectal cancer was observed to have high functional outcomes without any compromise in the oncological control (Bibas et al., 2022). In the management of prostate cancer, the nerve-sparing radical prostatectomy has helped in reducing post-treatment morbidity when compared to RT-related side effects. The side effects may be erectile dysfunction and urinary incontinence (Bauer et al., 2022).

AVOIDANCE OF RADIATION-RELATED TOXICITIES

RT is related to various long-term adverse effects like fibrosis, secondary malignancies and chronic organ dysfunction. The patients who undergo pelvic radiation therapy for rectal cancer may experience radiation proctitis and increased bowel dysfunction. Meanwhile, the surgical alternatives such as total mesorectal excision (TME) can provide some curative approach without any complications induced by radiation (AlEnazi et al., 2023). Also in head and neck cancers, the surgical excision that has a selective neck dissection decreases the xerostomia and osteoradionecrosis risks. These are the common post-RT complications (Wilson, 1984).

PATIENT SELECTION FOR NO-RT SURGICAL APPROACHES

Despite having many advantages not all tumours are amendable to the NO-RT surgical strategy. Factors like tumour size, invasion depth, nodal involvement and patient comorbidities must be carefully evaluated. Multidisciplinary tumours play an important role in determining patients' eligibility. This helps in ensuring that NO-RT surgery maintains oncologic efficacy and also improves the quality of life (Bibas et al., 2022). By combining the advanced surgical modalities, management of tumours can continue to evolve towards personalized and organ-preserving approaches, thus reducing the reliance on RT where possible.

The pivotal trials in rectal and breast cancer, such as the PROSPECT and CALGB 9343 trials, have significantly influenced treatment paradigms by comparing outcomes of surgery alone versus adjuvant RT. These trials aimed to assess the efficacy of neoadjuvant therapies and their impact on disease-free survival (DFS) and overall survival (OS), ultimately guiding clinical decision-making.

OVERVIEW OF KEY TRIALS

The PROSPECT trial, a phase 3 study, assessed the effectiveness of neoadjuvant folinic acid, fluorouracil and oxaliplatin (FOLFOX) chemotherapy with selective use of fluorouracil (5FU)-based chemoradiation compared to standard chemoradiotherapy in patients with locally advanced rectal cancer. The primary endpoint was DFS, with secondary endpoints including OS and local recurrence rates (Schrag et al., 2023). The CALGB 9343 trial focused on women aged 70 and older with early-stage oestrogen receptor-positive breast cancer. It evaluated whether adjuvant RT post-lumpectomy was necessary by comparing local recurrence and survival rates between surgery alone and surgery with RT (Felder et al., 2024). The IDEA trial investigated adjuvant chemotherapy duration in breast cancer, highlighting the need for personalized treatment strategies based on patient-specific risk factors (Hajibandeh & Hajibandeh, 2015). Emerging trials in head and neck cancer continue to explore RT omission in select patient groups based on molecular and clinical risk stratification.

METHODOLOGY

These trials employed rigorous inclusion and exclusion criteria. The PROSPECT trial included patients with T2/T3 node-positive or node-negative rectal cancer, excluding those with metastatic disease or poor performance status (Schrag et al., 2023). Similarly, CALGB 9343 enrolled elderly patients with T1–T2, N0, M0 breast cancer while excluding those with aggressive histology (Felder et al., 2024). The trials used statistical measures such as hazard ratios (HRs) and confidence intervals (CIs) to assess DFS and OS, with non-inferiority margins to determine treatment equivalence (Schrag et al., 2023).

RESULTS AND IMPLICATIONS

The PROSPECT trial demonstrated non-inferiority of neoadjuvant FOLFOX chemotherapy compared to chemoradiation, suggesting RT omission in selected rectal cancer patients (Schrag et al., 2023). CALGB 9343 found that omitting RT in elderly, low-risk breast cancer patients did not significantly affect OS but slightly increased local recurrence risk (Felder et al., 2024). Limitations of these studies included patient heterogeneity and limited follow-up duration, necessitating further research (Hajibandeh & Hajibandeh, 2015).

INTEGRATION INTO CLINICAL DECISION-MAKING

These trials have contributed to a paradigm shift towards NO-RT strategies in selected patients. Multidisciplinary teams increasingly integrate these findings into patient counselling, balancing oncologic safety with quality of life (Schrag et al., 2023; Felder et al., 2024). Ongoing trials aim to refine these strategies further (**Table 3.1**).

TABLE 3.1 Summary of Major Trials Informing NO-RT Strategies

Trial Name	Cancer Type	Patient Group	Key Findings
PROSPECT	Rectal cancer	Locally advanced	Neoadjuvant FOLFOX non-inferior to chemoradiation
CALGB 9343	Breast cancer	Elderly, early stage, ER+	Omitting RT had minimal impact on OS
IDEA	Breast cancer	Various risk groups	Emphasized personalized treatment strategies

WHEN IS SURGERY PREFERRED OVER RADIOTHERAPY?

Surgery is one of the frequently preferred treatment modalities over RT in specific clinical scenarios. This can be particularly useful when considering tumour characteristics, patient factors and potential long-term complications. The decision is generally guided by the anatomical location of the tumour, resectability, patient demographics and emerging molecular profiling techniques.

Localized and Resectable Tumours

For the tumours that are well localized and completely resectable, surgery can be considered as the optimal approach. In head and neck malignancies, one of the important factors that needs to be achieved is negative surgical margins. This is because local control influences the cervical outcomes of patients (Homer & Fardy, 2016). In paediatric oncology, surgical resection was preferred when necessary, as it helps in reducing the need for RT, which can be associated with growth abnormalities, neurocognitive deficits and secondary malignancies (Daya et al., 2000). Similarly, in some early-stage breast cancers and soft tissue sarcomas, priority will be given to complete excision so as to avoid the potential complications of RT (Dairo et al., 2024).

Avoiding Long-Term Toxicity of RT

RT may be effective, but there are risks of long-term adverse effects. This can be observed particularly in young patients and specific anatomical sites. Some of the toxicities caused by RT are fibrosis, secondary malignancies, endocrine dysfunction and neurocognitive impairments (Daya et al., 2000). In head and neck cancers, the usage of RT can lead to xerostomia, dysphagia and osteoradionecrosis. This may affect the quality of life of patients (Dairo et al., 2024). In these cases, surgery can be integrated with other reconstructive techniques like microvascular free flap reconstruction. This acts as an alternative that can maintain function and also helps in effective removal of tumours (Dairo et al., 2024).

Patient Preference and Genetic Resistance to RT

Autonomy of patients also plays a significant role in treatment decision-making. Some patients may choose to forego RT because of concerns about long-term toxicity. This can be observed particularly in young adults and those with a strong familial predisposition to radiation-induced malignancies (Homer & Fardy, 2016). Also, advancements in molecular profiling have identified genetic markers predictive of RT resistance. Tumours that show the radioresistant phenotypes, such as those with TP53 mutations or hypoxic microenvironments, may be removed completely by the surgical approach (Suárez et al., 2015).

KEY SURGICAL TECHNIQUES IN NO-RT

While surgery is preferred in localized, resectable tumours and cases where RT toxicity is a major concern, treatment decisions should be individualized. In scenarios where tumours are unresectable or highly radiosensitive, RT remains a valuable option. A multidisciplinary approach integrating surgical oncology, radiation oncology and molecular diagnostics is essential for optimizing patient outcomes. Minimally invasive surgery (MIS) has revolutionized oncology by improving surgical precision, reducing complications and facilitating faster recovery. Techniques such as laparoscopic and robotic-assisted surgeries have enabled effective cancer treatment while minimizing the need for RT. The following sections explore key surgical techniques in NO-RT.

Laparoscopic Surgery

Laparoscopic colectomy is a commonly adopted technique in colorectal cancer treatment. It mainly involves small incisions that result in reduced postoperative pain, faster recovery and lower complication rates compared to open surgery (Pathak & Wanjari, 2023). The laparoscopic surgery leads to decreased blood loss, shorter hospital stays and better long-term quality of life (Bakshi et al., 2024). Moreover, avoiding RT in rectal cancer patients through laparoscopic interventions prevents radiation-associated complications like bowel dysfunction and secondary malignancies (Pérez Ayme et al., 2023).

Robotic-Assisted Surgery

Robotic prostatectomy has become the standard of care for localized prostate cancer. This helped in eliminating the need for adjuvant RT in many cases (Waqas et al., 2022). The use of robotic platforms provides improved surgical precision, thus reducing the risk of complications like anastomotic leaks and nerve damage (Pérez Ayme et al., 2024). Advanced imaging techniques and robotic articulation help in nerve-sparing procedures, preserving urinary and sexual function and also ensuring oncological safety. Despite its advantages, MIS faces challenges like high costs, a steep learning curve and limited accessibility in certain regions. However, continuous technological advancements are expected to broaden the scope of MIS and improve patient outcomes globally (Pérez Ayme et al., 2023).

Organ-Sparing Surgery

Breast Cancer—Lumpectomy and Endocrine Therapy

Organ-sparing surgery in breast cancer as a lumpectomy combined with endocrine therapy (ET) has emerged as an effective alternative to whole-breast RT in selected hormone receptor-positive early-stage patients. It has been shown that older women ≥65 years with small, low-risk tumours can safely forgo RT when treated with ET, without compromising survival outcomes (Ortabaeva et al., 2022; Shen et al., 2023). The CALGB 9343 trial has also confirmed that the omission of RT in this subgroup does not significantly impact OS or distant metastasis rates (Hughes et al., 2013). However, adherence to ET remains critical because the patients who complete the full duration of treatment experience significantly reduced locoregional recurrence rates (Seol et al., 2022).

Bladder Cancer: TURBT and Chemotherapy

For bladder cancer, transurethral resection of the bladder tumour (TURBT) combined with chemotherapy can be an alternative to radical cystectomy. This can be particularly observed in patients with significant comorbidities or those unwilling to undergo major surgery (Niedworok et al., 2016). TURBT helps in effective tumour control while preserving bladder function, minimizing perioperative complications and improving the quality of life (Kim & Patel, 2020). However, careful patient selection is necessary because those with aggressive or recurrent disease may need more extensive interventions. Personalized treatment strategies like surveillance and adjuvant therapies are necessary for optimized outcomes.

Cytoreductive Surgery and Hyperthermic Intraperitoneal Chemotherapy in Advanced Ovarian Cancer

Cytoreductive surgery (CRS) followed by hyperthermic intraperitoneal chemotherapy (HIPEC) can be used as a therapeutic option for advanced ovarian cancer. This can be used in cases with extensive peritoneal carcinomatosis. HIPEC improves the delivery of chemotherapy by exposing residual tumour cells to heated chemotherapeutic agents, thus improving the penetration of the drug and cytotoxicity (Aronson et al., 2024). HIPEC can prolong progression-free survival and OS in patients undergoing interval CRS (Graham et al., 2024). However, its role in replacing postoperative RT remains inconclusive. While HIPEC may reduce tumour burden, recurrence rates are still comparable to CRS alone; this makes it necessary to individualize decisions on RT use (Imperio-Onglao & Luna, 2024). The integration of HIPEC into standard protocols is limited by variability in patient outcomes. This shows the need for further trials to determine its definitive impact on postoperative RT necessity (Mutlu Sütcüoğlu & Sütcüoğlu, 2023).

Sentinel Lymph Node Biopsy Instead of Full Lymph Node Dissection

Sentinel lymph node biopsy (SLNB) can be considered as a standard technique in breast cancer and melanoma surgeries. This helps in reducing the morbidity and also helps in accurate staging. Unlike axillary lymph node dissection (ALND), SLNB selectively identifies the first lymph nodes draining the tumour and minimizes unnecessary removal of uninvolved nodes (Gentile & Tinterri, 2024). SLNB also lowers the risk of complications such as lymphedema, pain and nerve injury compared to ALND (Espejo Niño, 2023). For many patients with positive sentinel nodes, omitting ALND does not compromise recurrence-free survival or OS (Sulthana & Singh, 2024). SLNB provides reliable staging in clinically node-negative patients and those undergoing neoadjuvant chemotherapy (Moushaly et al., 2023). The sentinel node identification rate is high, with studies reporting success rates around 95% (Espejo Niño, 2023). Despite its benefits, concerns remain regarding its use in patients with extra-nodal extension or micrometastases, necessitating further research (**Table 3.2**) (Moushaly et al., 2023).

TABLE 3.2 Surgery vs. Radiation: Decision Framework

Cancer Type	Surgical Alternative to RT	RT-Dependent Scenarios
Breast cancer (early-stage HR+)	Lumpectomy + Endocrine therapy	Triple-negative or HER2+ Tumours requiring RT
Prostate cancer (localized)	Radical prostatectomy	High-risk disease requiring adjuvant RT
NSCLC (stage I)	Lobectomy	Inoperable cases where SBRT is preferred
Rectal cancer (TNT approach)	Non-operative management (watch and wait)	Locally advanced requiring neoadjuvant RT
Ovarian cancer	CRS + HIPEC	Late-stage cases with high peritoneal spread

CASE STUDIES DEMONSTRATING NO-RT VIA SURGERY

The comparison of survival rates between the traditional approach of radiotherapy with surgery and surgery with No-RT in specific cancer groups—namely breast, lung, rectal and prostate cancer—is shown in **Figure 3.2**.

Case 1—Early-Stage Breast Cancer without Radiation

A 72-year-old female patient with hormone receptor-positive, low-risk early-stage breast cancer underwent lumpectomy followed by ET, omitting postoperative RT. This decision aligned with emerging evidence suggesting that older women with low-risk hormone receptor-positive breast cancer may not experience significant survival benefits from RT, despite a potential increase in local recurrence rates. In this case, the patient remained disease free for 5 years, with a disease-free survival rate of 94%. Notably, she avoided RT-related side effects such as skin toxicity, fatigue and potential cardiac complications. The case highlights the evolving approach to treatment de-escalation in elderly breast cancer patients, emphasizing personalized decision-making based on tumour biology, patient age and comorbidities. As studies continue to explore the long-term effects of omitting RT, clinicians are increasingly considering ET alone for select patients, balancing the risks of local recurrence with the benefits of reduced treatment burden and preserved quality of life (Bennett, 2021).

Neoadjuvant Chemotherapy for Locally Advanced Rectal Cancer

The PROSPECT trial (Alliance N1048) evaluated whether neoadjuvant chemotherapy alone (FOLFOX) could replace the standard approach of chemoradiation therapy (5FU CRT) in patients with locally advanced rectal cancer, reducing the need for RT. This approach aimed to spare patients the long-term morbidity of RT while maintaining oncological outcomes. Surgery played a crucial role in demonstrating the feasibility of this NO-RT strategy. Patients in the FOLFOX arm underwent rectal surgery after six cycles of chemotherapy, contingent on a tumour size reduction of at least 20%. If this response criterion was not met, patients proceeded to CRT before surgery. The surgical outcomes validated the efficacy of chemotherapy alone in many patients, allowing a subset to avoid RT entirely. Patient-reported outcomes (PROs) reinforced the benefits of this approach,

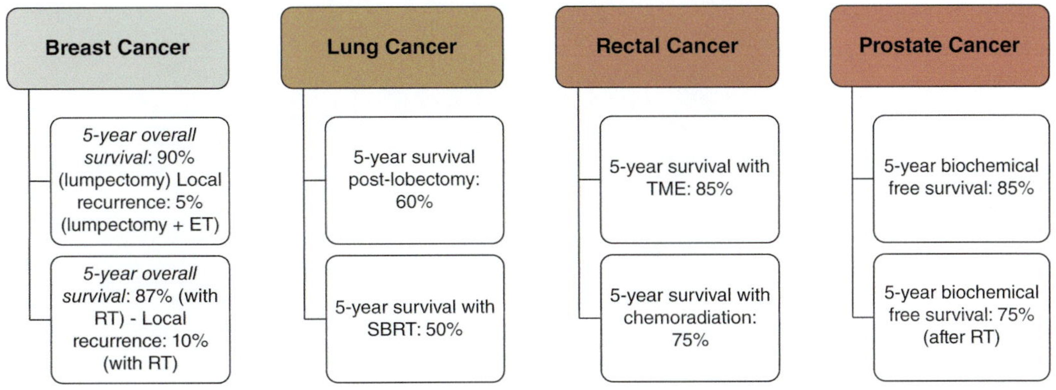

FIGURE 3.2 Surgical vs. radiation-based treatment outcomes in selected cancers.

with the FOLFOX group reporting lower rates of bowel dysfunction and neuropathy at 12 months post-surgery compared to the 5FU CRT group. These findings highlight the potential of surgery as a decisive factor in identifying patients who can forgo radiation without compromising treatment success.

The PROSPECT trial thus supports a selective approach, offering patients a personalized, less toxic treatment pathway (Basch et al., 2023).

Watch-and-Wait Strategy in Rectal Cancer

The concept of non-operative rectal tumour management (NO-RT) has gained traction with the emergence of watch-and-wait (WW) strategies for rectal cancer patients who achieve a clinical complete response (cCR) following neoadjuvant therapy. However, salvage surgery remains a critical component in cases where local regrowth occurs. The study by Smith et al. (2019) demonstrated that among 113 rectal cancer patients managed via WW, 22 (19%) experienced local regrowth, all of whom underwent successful salvage surgery. TME was the primary surgical approach, with 91% achieving pelvic tumour control post-surgery. This evidence highlights that NO-RT through WW is feasible in selected patients, with a high rate of organ preservation (82%). However, the study also underscores the importance of vigilant monitoring, as patients with local regrowth had a higher incidence of distant metastases (36% vs. 1%). While NO-RT reduces the morbidity associated with radical surgery, it necessitates precise patient selection and close follow-up to ensure timely intervention when necessary. These findings suggest that while WW strategies contribute to rectal preservation, salvage surgery remains essential for achieving optimal oncologic outcomes in cases of tumour recurrence.

The stepwise clinical decision-making guidance process for determining when to use radiotherapy versus when to consider a No-RT approach across various cancer types is outlined in **Figure 3.3**. and **Table 3.3**.

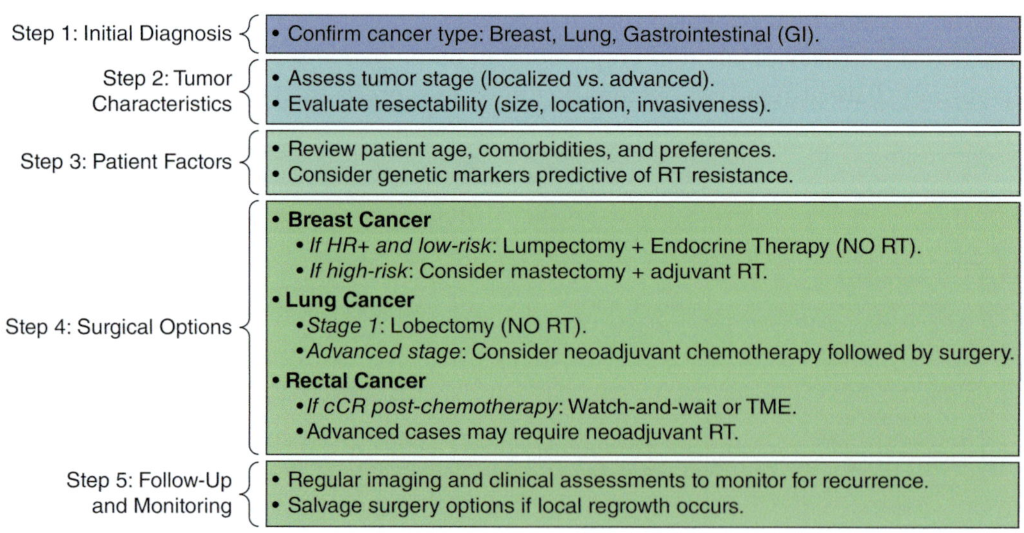

FIGURE 3.3 Decision Guidance Tree for NO-RT via surgery in breast, lung and rectal cancers.

TABLE 3.3 Biomarkers that Support RT Omission

Biomarker	Cancer Type	Clinical Relevance	Impact on RT Decision	Supporting Study/Trial
Oestrogen receptor (ER)	Breast cancer	High ER expression indicates hormone responsiveness	High ER+ tumours in elderly patients can safely omit RT with endocrine therapy	CALGB 9343 Hughes et al., 2013
Progesterone receptor (PR)	Breast cancer	PR positivity strengthens hormonal responsiveness	Supports RT omission in combination with ER+ and endocrine therapy	CALGB 9343 Shen et al., 2023
Ki-67 (<13%)	Breast cancer	Indicates low proliferation index	Lower risk of recurrence allows consideration for RT omission	Seol et al., 2022
Oncotype DX Recurrence Score (RS <18)	Breast cancer	Assesses recurrence risk in ER+/HER2− cancers	Low RS supports omitting RT in low-risk patients on endocrine therapy	Sparano et al., 2015
TP53 wild-type	Multiple	Functional p53 linked to RT sensitivity	Wild-type may not predict RT resistance, but mutations support surgery focus	Suárez et al., 2015
HPV-positivity	Head and neck SCC	Indicates better prognosis and radiosensitivity	In select cases, supports de-escalation or omission of RT	Gillison et al., 2019
Mucinous histology	Colorectal cancer	Associated with favourable prognosis	Potential candidate for NO-RT approaches after resection	Dairo et al., 2024
Microsatellite stability (MSS)	Colorectal cancer	Lower immunogenicity than MSI-H tumours	More predictable response to surgery; RT may be avoided	Pérez Ayme et al., 2023

REAL-WORLD CASE STUDY

Mrs. L's case exemplifies a growing trend in personalized breast cancer care, where adjuvant RT can be safely omitted in carefully selected older patients with favourable tumour biology.

Clinical Justification

The decision to forgo RT in Mrs. L's treatment plan is supported by several key studies:

- **CALGB 9343 Trial**: This pivotal study demonstrated that women aged 70 and older with stage 1 oestrogen receptor (ER)-positive breast cancer who underwent lumpectomy and received tamoxifen had a low risk of locoregional recurrence, even without RT. The 10-year local recurrence rate was 10% without RT compared to 2% with RT, with no significant difference in OS between the groups (Hughes et al., 2004).
- **PRIME II Trial**: This study found that women aged 65 and older with hormone receptor-positive, node-negative breast cancer who received ET after breast-conserving surgery had a low risk of local recurrence without RT. The omission of RT did not adversely affect OS (Ho & Bellon, 2023; Kunkler et al., 2023).
- **IDEA Trial**: This research extended the findings to younger postmenopausal women (aged 50–69) with low-risk, ER/progesterone receptor (PR)-positive, HER2-negative tumours and low Oncotype DX Recurrence Scores (≤18). The 5-year freedom from any recurrence was 99%, suggesting that RT omission is safe in this broader age group when combined with ET (Jagsi et al., 2024).

Patient-Centred Outcomes

At her 5-year follow-up, Mrs. L remained free of local recurrence and reported excellent quality of life, highlighting the benefits of individualized treatment strategies that minimize unnecessary interventions. Mrs. L's case underscores the importance of tailoring breast cancer treatment based on patient age, tumour biology and genomic risk assessments. By integrating clinical trial evidence into practice, clinicians can make informed decisions that prioritize patient wellbeing without compromising outcomes.

CONCLUSION

This chapter underscores the critical role of surgery in tumour management, particularly as a viable alternative to RT in select cases. Advances in minimally invasive techniques, robotic-assisted procedures and organ-sparing surgeries have significantly enhanced oncologic outcomes while reducing treatment-related morbidities. By prioritizing precise tumour excision, these surgical innovations enable improved local control, minimize recurrence risks and mitigate long-term toxicities commonly associated with RT. Surgery remains the preferred approach in patients with localized, resectable tumours where complete excision can provide curative potential. Techniques such as laparoscopic colectomy, robotic prostatectomy and TaTME exemplify how surgical strategies can effectively replace RT, particularly in cases where preserving organ function and quality of life are paramount. Additionally, organ-sparing procedures, including lumpectomy with endocrine therapy for breast cancer and TURBT for bladder cancer, offer viable alternatives to traditional RT regimens.

CRS with HIPEC further exemplifies the potential of surgical advancements in reducing the need for RT in advanced malignancies. Despite these advantages, patient selection remains crucial, necessitating a multidisciplinary approach to tailor treatment strategies based on tumour characteristics, molecular profiles and patient preferences. Future research should focus on refining surgical techniques, integrating novel imaging modalities and enhancing precision oncology to expand the scope of NO-RT treatment paradigms. As surgical oncology continues to evolve, its role in reducing reliance on RT while maintaining oncologic efficacy will remain integral to optimizing patient outcomes in cancer care.

REFERENCES

AlEnazi, N., Alanazi, A. Q., Al-Rabia, M. W., & Albisi, F. (2023). Treatment of cancer. In F. Q. B. Alenzi (Ed.), *Molecular Targets and Cancer Therapeutics (Part 2)* (pp. 122–164). Bentham Science Publishers. https://doi.org/10.2174/9789815124606123010006

Aronson, S. L., Lopez-Yurda, M., Koole, S. N., Schagen Van Leeuwen, J. H., Schreuder, H. W. R., Hermans, R. H. M., De Hingh, I. H. J. T., Van Gent, M. D. J. M., Arts, H. J. G., Van Ham, M. A. P. C., Van Dam, P. A., Vuylsteke, P., Aalbers, A. G. J., Verwaal, V. J., Van De Vijver, K. K., Aaronson, N. K., Sonke, G. S., & Van Driel, W. J. (2024). Cytoreductive surgery with or without hyperthermic intraperitoneal chemotherapy in patients with advanced ovarian cancer (OVHIPEC-1): Final survival analysis of a randomised, controlled, phase 3 trial. *Obstetrical & Gynecological Survey, 79*(2), 96–98. https://doi.org/10.1097/01.ogx.0001008536.08634.9f

Bakshi, I., Rana, P., Srivastava, G., & Rawat, H. S. (2024). Comparing minimally invasive techniques to traditional surgery for specific tumor or cancer types: A comprehensive review. *International Journal For Multidisciplinary Research*, *6*(2), 14944. https://doi.org/10.36948/ijfmr.2024.v06i02.14944

Basch, E., Dueck, A. C., Mitchell, S. A., Mamon, H., Weiser, M., Saltz, L., Gollub, M., Rogak, L., Ginos, B., Mazza, G. L., Colgrove, B., Chang, G., Minasian, L., Denicoff, A., Thanarajasingam, G., Musher, B., George, T., Venook, A., Farma, J., O'Reilly, E., Meyerhardt, J. A., Shi, Q., & Schrag, D. (2023). Patient-reported outcomes during and after treatment for locally advanced rectal cancer in the PROSPECT trial (Alliance N1048). *Journal of Clinical Oncology*, *41*(21), 3724–3734. https://doi.org/10.1200/JCO.23.00903

Bauer, T. W., Tanabe, K. K., & Pollock, R. E. (2022). Principles of surgical oncology. In R. C. Bast, W. N. Hait, D. W. Kufe, R. R. Weichselbaum, J. F. Holland, C. M. Croce, M. Piccart-Gebart, H. Wang, W. K. Hong & R. E. Pollock (Eds.), *Holland-Frei Cancer Medicine* (1st ed., pp. 1–12). Wiley. https://doi.org/10.1002/9781119000822.hfcm044.pub2

Bennett, B. (2021). A closure look on benefits of radiation therapy. *Journal of Cancer Science & Therapy*, *12*, 428.

Bibas, I. D. F. P., Ross, F. S., Morila, M. C. G., Neto, R. P., Lima, J. H. C. D., Gunther, M. G., Karvat, J. G. V., Magalhães, M. C. F., & Preti, V. B. (2022). Surgical approaches and techniques in cancer treatment: Past, present, and future/Abordagens e técnicas cirúrgicas no tratamento oncológico: Passado, presente e futuro. *Brazilian Journal of Health Review*, *5*(2), 7196–7213. https://doi.org/10.34119/bjhrv5n2-280

Dairo, K., Bishop, R., Sethia, R., Old, M., Jatana, K. R., & Elmaraghy, C. A. (2024). Local control of pediatric head and neck sarcoma with free flap reconstruction obviating the need for radiotherapy: A case report. *Translational Pediatrics*, *13*(8), 1503–1509. https://doi.org/10.21037/tp-24-4

Daya, H., Chan, H. S. L., Sirkin, W., & Forte, V. (2000). Pediatric rhabdomyosarcoma of the head and neck: Is there a place for surgical management? *Archives of Otolaryngology–Head & Neck Surgery*, *126*(4), 468. https://doi.org/10.1001/archotol.126.4.468

Espejo Niño, J. M. (2023). 367P Sentinel lymph node biopsy (SLNB) in patients with locally advanced breast cancer (LABC): Descriptive, inferential and survival analysis. *Annals of Oncology*, *34*, S329. https://doi.org/10.1016/j.annonc.2023.09.545

Felder, S., Frakes, J., George, M., Rosen, A., & Sahin, I. H. (2024). Which treatment for which patient: Rectal cancer management after PROSPECT trial. *Oncology*, *38*(5), 187–190. https://doi.org/10.46883/2024.25921019

Gentile, D., & Tinterri, C. (2024). Sentinel lymph node biopsy versus axillary lymph node dissection in breast cancer patients undergoing mastectomy. *Minerva Surgery*, *79*(5). https://doi.org/10.23736/S2724-5691.24.10485-6

Gillison, M. L., Trotti, A. M., Harris, J., Eisbruch, A., Harari, P. M., Adelstein, D. J., … & RTOG 1016 Investigators. (2019). Radiotherapy plus cetuximab or cisplatin in human papillomavirus–positive oropharyngeal cancer (RTOG 1016): A randomised, multicentre, non-inferiority trial. *Lancet*, 393(10166), 51–60. https://doi.org/10.1016/S0140-6736(18)32779-X.

Graham, R., MacDonald, N. D., Mould, T. A., & Kotsopoulos, I. C. (2024). Hyperthermic intraperitoneal chemotherapy (HIPEC) in the management of ovarian cancer. *Obstetrician & Gynaecologist*, *26*(2), 76–83. https://doi.org/10.1111/tog.12916

Hajibandeh, S., & Hajibandeh, S. (2015). Systematic review: Adjuvant chemotherapy for locally advanced rectal cancer with respect to stage of disease. *International Scholarly Research Notices*, *2015*, 1–10. https://doi.org/10.1155/2015/710569

Ho, A. Y., & Bellon, J. R. (2023). Overcoming resistance—Omission of radiotherapy for low-risk breast cancer. *New England Journal of Medicine*, *388*(7), 652–653. https://doi.org/10.1056/NEJMe2216133

Homer, J. J., & Fardy, M. J. (2016). Surgery in head and neck cancer: United Kingdom national multidisciplinary guidelines. *Journal of Laryngology & Otology*, *130*(S2), S68–S70. https://doi.org/10.1017/S0022215116000475

Hughes, K. S., Schnaper, L. A., Bellon, J. R., Cirrincione, C. T., Berry, D. A., McCormick, B., Muss, H. B., Smith, B. L., Hudis, C. A., Winer, E. P., & Wood, W. C. (2013). Lumpectomy plus tamoxifen with or without irradiation in women age 70 years or older with early breast cancer: Long-term follow-up of CALGB 9343. *Journal of Clinical Oncology, 31*(19), 2382–2387. https://doi.org/10.1200/JCO.2012.45.2615

Hughes, K. S., Schnaper, L. A., Berry, D., Cirrincione, C., McCormick, B., Shank, B., Wheeler, J., Champion, L. A., Smith, T. J., Smith, B. L., Shapiro, C., Muss, H. B., Winer, E., Hudis, C., Wood, W., Sugarbaker, D., Henderson, I. C., & Norton, L. (2004). Lumpectomy plus tamoxifen with or without irradiation in women 70 years of age or older with early breast cancer. *New England Journal of Medicine, 351*(10), 971–977. https://doi.org/10.1056/NEJMoa040587

Imperio-Onglao, R. A. P., & Luna (2024). Effect of cytoreductive surgery and hyperthermic intraperitoneal chemotherapy on epithelial ovarian, fallopian tube, and peritoneal cancer: An institutional review of outcomes and its clinical implications. *Philippine Journal of Obstetrics and Gynecology, 48*(1), 10–21. https://doi.org/10.4103/pjog.pjog_73_23

Jagsi, R., Griffith, K. A., Harris, E. E., Wright, J. L., Recht, A., Taghian, A. G., Lee, L., Moran, M. S., Small, W., Johnstone, C., Rahimi, A., Freedman, G., Muzaffar, M., Haffty, B., Horst, K., Powell, S. N., Sharp, J., Sabel, M., Schott, A., & El-Tamer, M. (2024). Omission of radiotherapy after breast-conserving surgery for women with breast cancer with low clinical and genomic risk: 5-year outcomes of IDEA. *Journal of Clinical Oncology, 42*(4), 390–398. https://doi.org/10.1200/JCO.23.02270

Kim, L. H. C., & Patel, M. I. (2020). Transurethral resection of bladder tumour (TURBT). *Translational Andrology and Urology, 9*(6), 3056–3072. https://doi.org/10.21037/tau.2019.09.38

Kunkler, I. H., Williams, L. J., Jack, W. J. L., Cameron, D. A., & Dixon, J. M. (2023). Breast-conserving surgery with or without irradiation in early breast cancer. *New England Journal of Medicine, 388*(7), 585–594. https://doi.org/10.1056/NEJMoa2207586

Moushaly, R. A., Ion, D., Andronic, O., Socea, B., Palcau, A. C., & Păduraru, D. N. (2023). Sentinel node biopsy for personalized breast cancer management: Advances and controversies. *Journal of Mind and Medical Sciences, 10*(2), 247–253. https://doi.org/10.22543/2392-7674.1440

Mutlu Sütcüoğlu, B., & Sütcüoğlu, O. (2023). Cytoreductive surgery with or without hyperthermic intraperitoneal chemotherapy in advanced ovarian cancer. *Lancet Oncology, 24*(12), e457. https://doi.org/10.1016/S1470-2045(23)00471-0

Niedworok, C., Shaleva, A., Rübben, H., & Stenzl, A. (2016). Organerhaltende therapie des harnblasenkarzinoms. *Der Urologe, 55*(5), 609–614. https://doi.org/10.1007/s00120-016-0086-5

Ortabaeva, D. R., Zikiryakhodzhaev, A. D., Rasskazova, E. A., Saribekyan, E. K., & Kaprin, A. D. (2022). Long-term oncological outcomes of organ-sparing treatment of patients with early breast cancer aged 65 years and older who had no postoperative radiation therapy. *Tumors of Female Reproductive System, 18*(3), 24–28. https://doi.org/10.17650/1994-4098-2022-18-3-24-28

Pathak, A., & Wanjari, M. (2023). Minimally invasive colorectal surgery techniques. *Cureus*. https://doi.org/10.7759/cureus.47203

Pérez Ayme, A. P., Caiza Suárez, J. M., Paredes Ortega, M. M., Gualoto Gualoto, D. S., Santillán Lima, J. C., Rivera Campoverde, A. E., Rivera Ticona, A. A., Coello Vergara, J. S., & Martínez Serrano, G. D. (2023). Advancements in minimally invasive surgical techniques: A comprehensive review. *Salud, Ciencia y Tecnología - Serie de Conferencias, 2*, 622. https://doi.org/10.56294/sctconf2023622

Pérez Ayme, A. P., Caiza Suárez, J. M., Paredes Ortega, M. M., Gualoto Gualoto, G. G., Santillán Lima, S. L., Rivera Campoverde, A. E., Rivera Ticona, A. A., Coello Vergara, C. V., & Martínez Serrano, G. D. (2024). Advancements in minimally invasive surgical techniques: A comprehensive review. *Salud, Ciencia y Tecnología, 3*, 745. https://doi.org/10.56294/saludcyt2023745

Schrag, D., Shi, Q., Weiser, M. R., Gollub, M. J., Saltz, L. B., Musher, B. L., Goldberg, J., Al Baghdadi, T., Goodman, K. A., McWilliams, R. R., Farma, J. M., George, T. J., Kennecke, H. F., Venook, A. P., O'Reilly, E. M., Meyerhardt, J. A., Dueck, A. C., Basch, E., ... Chang, G. J. (2023). PROSPECT: A randomized phase III trial of neoadjuvant chemoradiation versus neoadjuvant FOLFOX chemotherapy with selective use of chemoradiation, followed by total mesorectal excision (TME) for treatment of locally advanced rectal cancer (LARC) (Alliance n1048). *Journal of Clinical Oncology, 41*(17_suppl), LBA2. https://doi.org/10.1200/JCO.2023.41.17_suppl.LBA2

Seol, S. W., Pflederer, T., Weller, L., Goodman, C., Donnelly, E. D., Hayes, J. P., & Strauss, J. B. (2022). Abstract P1-13-03: Radiotherapy vs. endocrine therapy for hormone receptor positive early stage breast cancer accounting for endocrine therapy adherence. *Cancer Research, 82*(4_Supplement), P1-13-03-P1-13–03. https://doi.org/10.1158/1538-7445.SABCS21-P1-13-03

Shen, C., Li, N., Zhou, S., Stahl, K., Dodge, D., & Zhao, H. (2023). Endocrine therapy initiation and overall survival outcomes with omission of radiation therapy in older Medicare patients with early-stage hormone-receptor-positive breast cancer. *Cancer Medicine, 12*(6), 6935–6944. https://doi.org/10.1002/cam4.5488

Smith, J. J., Strombom, P., Chow, O. S., Roxburgh, C. S., Lynn, P., Eaton, A., Widmar, M., Ganesh, K., Yaeger, R., Cercek, A., Weiser, M. R., Nash, G. M., Guillem, J. G., Temple, L. K. F., Chalasani, S. B., Fuqua, J. L., Petkovska, I., Wu, A. J., Reyngold, M., ... Paty, P. B. (2019). Assessment of a watch-and-wait strategy for rectal cancer in patients with a complete response after neoadjuvant therapy. *JAMA Oncology, 5*(4), e185896. https://doi.org/10.1001/jamaoncol.2018.5896

Sparano, J. A., Gray, R., Makower, D. F., Pritchard, K. I., Albain, K. S., Hayes, D. F., Geyer, C. E., Dees, E. C., & Paik, S. (2015). Prospective validation of a 21-gene expression assay in breast cancer. *New England Journal of Medicine, 373*(21), 2005–2014. https://doi.org/10.1056/NEJMoa1510764

Suárez, C., Takes, R. P., Silver, C. E., Rodrigo, J. P., Strojan, P., Woolgar, J. A., Haigentz, M., Hakan Coskun, H., De Bree, R., Owen, R. P., Elsheikh, M. N., Shaha, A. R., Rinaldo, A., & Ferlito, A. (2015). When is surgical therapy for head and neck malignant epithelial tumors not indicated? *European Archives of Oto-Rhino-Laryngology, 272*(3), 513–516. https://doi.org/10.1007/s00405-014-2895-8

Sulthana, R., & Singh, A. (2024). Is sentinel lymph node biopsy a viable alternative to axillary lymph node dissection in breast carcinoma patients who have received neo- adjuvant chemotherapy? *Cureus*. https://doi.org/10.7759/cureus.52698

Waqas, A., Mykoniatis, I., Sidiqi, N., Ahmed, A., Stefan, S., Naqvi, S., Harper, M., & Khan, J. (2022). Early experience of undertaking robotic assisted total mesorectal excision in rectal resections, avoiding a diverting stoma: Key enhancement of the anastomosis for no stoma technique — A case series. *Surgical Innovation, 30*(2), 158–165. https://doi.org/10.1177/15533506221108833

Wilson, R. E. (1984). Surgical oncology. *Cancer, 54*(S2), 2595–2598. https://doi.org/10.1002/1097-0142(19841201)54:2+<2595::AID-CNCR2820541402≥3.0.CO;2-0

CHAPTER 4

Alternative Modalities

Assessing Treatment Choices Other Than Radiation

Peeyush Shukla, Rahul Sapate and Sandeep Ishi

INTRODUCTION

Radiation therapy (RT) is commonly used in cancer treatment and helps in significantly advancing patient outcomes. However, it has some limitations that make it necessary to explore alternative approaches. This chapter provides details regarding systemic therapies, emerging technologies and patient-centred care strategies by highlighting innovative solutions to challenges in cancer management.

Despite technological advancements, RT faces constraints in efficacy for treating advanced cancers such as ovarian and pancreatic cancer, and here the survival rates remain stagnant (Allen et al., 2013). Toxicity is another significant issue in the cases of re-irradiated areas. This complicates the treatment of recurrent locoregional disease (Shukla & Bansal, 2015). Furthermore, factors like tumour hypoxia and inherent radioresistance also limit its effectiveness. This shows the need for novel approaches to improve tumour sensitivity (Kinsella, 1981; Shukla & Bansal, 2015). Systemic therapies, including targeted treatments and immunotherapy, address systemic diseases and improve outcomes (Allen et al., 2013). Advances like stereotactic body radiotherapy and proton therapy can reduce toxicity while improving tumour control (Kinsella, 1981; Van Houtte et al., 2021). Collaborative and multidisciplinary approaches that combine systemic therapies, surgery and advanced radiation techniques are essential for cases like head and neck cancers (Shukla & Bansal, 2015).

SYSTEMIC THERAPIES—ROLE OF CHEMOTHERAPY, IMMUNOTHERAPY AND TARGETED THERAPIES AS ALTERNATIVES TO RT

Chemotherapy

Chemotherapy is a systemic therapy that is an alternative to RT in the treatment of different kinds of cancers, mainly when the RT has limited efficacy. With the help of cytotoxic agents, chemotherapy targets rapidly dividing cells, including cancerous cells, and disrupts

DOI: 10.1201/9781003529071-4

their DNA synthesis and cell division processes. Commonly used drugs were platinum-based agents like cisplatin, taxanes like paclitaxel and anthracyclines like doxorubicin, which are frequently combined with targeted therapies for improved outcomes (Michaels et al., 2016; Tiefenbacher & Pirker, 2018).

Chemotherapy Operates through Two Primary Mechanisms

Cytotoxic Effects—The Drugs Inhibit Cell Proliferation and Induce Apoptosis in Malignant Cells

Targeted Therapies: Advanced approaches leverage molecular markers to target specific cancer cell characteristics, reducing damage to normal tissues and enhancing efficacy (Min & Lee, 2022).

Chemotherapy provides advantages over RT, including its systemic reach, by enabling the treatment of metastatic cancer and its potential for combination with other modalities to optimize outcomes (Hanna et al., 2017). However, significant limitations, such as severe side effects like nausea, fatigue and immunosuppression, are still present. Additionally, chemotherapy is less effective for localized tumours, whereas RT may provide more targeted benefits (Min & Lee, 2022).

Indications for Specific Cancers

- **Breast Cancer**: Chemotherapy is prioritized in aggressive subtypes, such as triple-negative breast cancer, where RT alone may be insufficient (Michaels et al., 2016).
- **Non-Small Cell Lung Cancer (NSCLC)**: In advanced stages, chemotherapy serves as a first-line treatment that is often combined with immunotherapy (Hanna et al., 2017).
- **Osteosarcoma**: Chemotherapy remains the cornerstone of treatment, particularly in managing metastasis. RT is less effective regarding this malignancy (Gazouli et al., 2021).

While chemotherapy provides an essential alternative to RT, its application requires a tailored, patient-centric approach to maximize benefits and mitigate adverse effects. Advances in combination therapies and targeted treatments continue to enhance its role in modern oncology.

EMERGING TECHNOLOGIES

Some emerging technologies in cancer treatment are focused ultrasound (FUS), radiofrequency ablation and proton therapy. These methods are helping to transform the landscape of oncology. These treatment methods provide an alternative to traditional RTs that help improve clinical outcomes, reduce adverse effects and preserve patients' quality of life. By using the mechanisms and technologies of this method, there may be significant morbidity reduction, precision improvement and the ability to target tumours more effectively.

FOCUSED ULTRASOUND

High-intensity focused ultrasound (HIFU) is a non-invasive treatment method mainly using focused sound waves to produce heat. Then it ablates tumours with minimal damage to surrounding tissues (Avedian et al., 2016; Panzone et al., 2022). The precise delivery of thermal energy through FUS helps in effective localized tumour treatment without a need for incisions or radiation. This method is highly effective in treating cancers like prostate or kidney. There are studies that show a biochemical survival rate of 75% at 5 years for prostate cancer patients (Blana et al., 2008). The non-invasive nature of this method helps reduce the risk of complications compared to traditional surgery. It also provides the potential for improved drug delivery, particularly when integrated with chemotherapy, thus improving the overall therapeutic effects (Panzone et al., 2022). HIFU's ability to precisely target tumour cells is a promising option for many patients as the health of the surrounding cells will be preserved. This can act as an alternative for those who prefer non-invasive methods.

RADIOFREQUENCY ABLATION

Radiofrequency (RF) ablation is another minimally invasive technique that can effectively treat organ-conflicted tumours. This is especially seen in the cases of renal cell carcinoma (Gallego Vilar et al., 2010). This method uses electric current to produce heat, and RF ablation induces coagulation necrosis in the tumour. This will lead to its destruction. This method has shown some favourable outcomes, which makes it a suitable alternative to traditional surgery for patients with small renal tumours. The main advantage of RF ablation is its ability to treat tumours without needing a large incision or more recovery time. This procedure can be carried out with the help of image guidance. This helps ensure precision in targeting the tumours and reduces injury to nearby tissues. This method allows patients to avoid more significant risks related to conventional surgeries like bleeding, infections and prolonged recovery periods (Gallego Vilar et al., 2010).

PROTON THERAPY

Proton therapy is one of the advanced forms of RT that mainly uses protons instead of traditional X-rays to treat different types of cancers. This treatment method has advantages for cancers near critical structures because the protons can precisely target these tissues and reduce damage to the surrounding healthy tissues. It has shown some significant improvement in treating non-prostate genitourinary cancers such as testicular tumours, bladder cancer and renal pelvis tumours. This method has an efficacy range of 90%–95% for specific cancer types (Cohen et al., 2022). The precision of proton therapy is an important factor in its effectiveness. Protons have unique physical properties called Bragg peaks that can help them deposit most of their energy directly into the tumour, unlike traditional radiation, which causes collateral damage to the surrounding tissue. This leads to better control and also reduces the impact on healthy tissues. This makes proton therapy more beneficial for paediatric patients and patients with complex or recurrent cancers (Chu, 1995). The technological advancements in proton therapy include the introduction of pencil beam scanning and advanced dose delivery methods. These have significantly improved the accuracy of the treatment. These improvements help with better tumour delineation and more effective treatment plans, thus helping reduce potential side effects and increasing the precision of tumour targeting (Schippers & Lomax, 2011). Also, the ongoing research in proton therapy mainly aims to improve the treatment delivery systems by integrating real-time imaging and developing smaller cyclotrons to create more accessible and compact treatment facilities (Schippers & Lomax, 2011). The high cost and the need for specialized infrastructure continue to be challenges to its widespread adoption, mainly in regions with limited healthcare resources.

Emerging technologies like FUS, RF ablation and proton therapy are revolutionizing cancer treatment. These methods provide significant advantages over traditional treatment methods, including reduced morbidity, improved precision and patient outcomes. As these technologies continue to evolve, these treatment options can become the standard practice in oncology and provide patients with a less invasive and more effective alternative to traditional RT. There are some challenges, such as high cost, accessibility and need for specialized facilities, that must be addressed to ensure that these treatment methods can reach a broader population of cancer patients.

EXAMPLES OF PATIENT OUTCOMES USING ALTERNATIVE MODALITIES

Histotripsy for Liver Cancer

Histotripsy, a non-invasive ultrasound-based technique, has shown promise in treating liver cancer. A patient with recurrent hepatocellular carcinoma (HCC) underwent histotripsy, achieving complete tumour ablation with minimal side effects. Unlike conventional treatments such as surgical resection, RF ablation or transarterial chemoembolization (TACE), histotripsy offers a precise and targeted approach with reduced damage to surrounding tissues. The patient's post-treatment imaging revealed no residual tumour activity, and follow-up assessments indicated a positive response with no recurrence for over a year. This case highlights histotripsy's potential as a viable alternative to traditional liver cancer therapies (Parashar et al., 2024).

Chemotherapy and Complementary and Alternative Medicine for Gastric Cancer

A patient diagnosed with advanced gastric cancer incorporated complementary and alternative medicine (CAM) into their treatment regimen alongside conventional chemotherapy. The CAM approach included acupuncture, herbal supplements and mind–body therapy to enhance overall wellbeing and immune response. Remarkably, the patient achieved complete remission and has remained cancer-free for over 9 years. This case underscores the potential benefits of integrating CAM with standard treatments to improve long-term patient outcomes. Personalized treatment strategies that consider both conventional and alternative approaches may contribute to improved survival rates and quality of life in cancer patients (Q & Q, 2015).

HIFU for Prostate Cancer

HIFU has gained recognition as a non-invasive treatment option for localized prostate cancer. A clinical study involving a cohort of prostate cancer patients reported a 5-year biochemical survival rate of 75% following HIFU treatment. The procedure effectively targeted and ablated cancerous tissue while preserving surrounding structures, reducing the risk of complications such as incontinence and erectile dysfunction. These outcomes suggest that HIFU can serve as a viable alternative to radical prostatectomy or RT, particularly for patients seeking a minimally invasive option with reduced side effects (Blana et al., 2008).

Nutritional Support in Breast Cancer Treatment

Nutritional interventions have been increasingly recognized for their role in cancer treatment outcomes. A patient with metastatic breast cancer underwent chemotherapy combined with a structured nutritional support programme designed to optimize immune function and reduce treatment-related toxicities. This personalized nutrition plan included a high-antioxidant diet, omega-3 supplementation and probiotic therapy. After completing chemotherapy, the patient achieved complete remission and remained disease-free for nearly 3 years. This case emphasizes the critical role of diet and nutrition in enhancing therapeutic efficacy, reducing adverse effects and improving overall quality of life in cancer patients (Taxman et al., 2016).

COMPARATIVE EFFECTIVENESS—THE EFFECTIVENESS OF ALTERNATIVES COMPARED TO RT

While RT remains a cornerstone in cancer treatment, its limitations in terms of efficacy and toxicity highlight the need for alternative approaches. The persistent challenges in treating advanced cancers such as ovarian and pancreatic cancer, as well as the complications in re-irradiating areas, underscore the importance of exploring other modalities. Emerging treatments like RF ablation, proton therapy and FUS are promising alternatives to RT, providing benefits such as reduced morbidity, improved precision and improved patient outcomes.

RF ablation is a minimally invasive procedure used primarily to treat organ-confined tumours, especially in renal cell carcinoma and liver metastases (Gallego Vilar et al., 2010). RF ablation uses electrical currents to generate heat, inducing coagulation necrosis in tumour tissues. The procedure can be performed percutaneously under imaging guidance, ensuring targeted therapy while minimizing damage to surrounding tissues. Compared to traditional surgery, RF ablation significantly reduces recovery time, risks of infection and complications such as bleeding (Gallego Vilar et al., 2010). Its non-invasive nature makes it an attractive option for patients seeking alternatives to conventional treatments. RF ablation is particularly effective for smaller tumours but may face limitations with larger or more complex masses. While RT provides higher precision in treating deeper or larger tumours, RF ablation is increasingly integrated into personalized treatment plans for patients with localized cancers, providing a safer and more efficient option when surgery is not feasible.

Proton therapy, an advanced form of radiation, uses protons instead of X-rays to treat various cancers. One of the significant advantages of proton therapy is its precision in delivering radiation, which minimizes collateral damage to surrounding healthy tissues, making it ideal for tumours near critical structures, such as in paediatric cases (Cohen et al., 2022). Unlike traditional RT, which spreads radiation beyond the tumour, proton therapy's unique physical property, the Bragg peak, ensures that most radiation is deposited directly within the tumour (Chu, 1995). Proton therapy has successfully treated paediatric brain tumours, head and neck cancers and genitourinary tumours, with efficacy rates ranging from 90% to 95% for specific cancer types (Cohen et al., 2022). However, the high cost and limited availability of proton therapy facilities present challenges to its widespread adoption. As advancements in treatment delivery methods, such as pencil beam scanning, improve precision, proton therapy is expected to play an increasingly critical role in personalized cancer treatment.

HIFU is another non-invasive technique that uses focused sound waves to generate heat and ablate tumours. Its precision in targeting tumours while preserving healthy tissue makes it a promising alternative to surgery and RT, particularly for prostate and kidney cancers (Avedian et al., 2016; Panzone et al., 2022). Studies show that HIFU offers long-term survival benefits, including a 5-year biochemical survival rate of 75% for prostate cancer patients (Blana et al., 2008). HIFU's significant advantages include reduced recovery times and the absence of incisions, making it a less invasive and safer alternative to traditional treatments. It also holds potential for enhancing drug delivery, particularly when combined with chemotherapy, further improving treatment outcomes (Panzone et al., 2022). However, HIFU's efficacy may be limited for tumours located deep within the body or those inaccessible via ultrasound.

Emerging treatment modalities such as RF ablation, proton therapy and HIFU represent significant advancements in cancer care. These therapies offer the potential to enhance precision, reduce toxicity and provide alternative options for patients who may not be suitable candidates for traditional RTs. However, the challenges of cost, accessibility and the need for specialized equipment must be addressed to ensure these alternatives are widely available. As research continues, these innovative treatments may become standard options in oncology, providing patients with more targeted, less invasive choices that improve overall survival and quality of life.

PATIENT-CENTRED CARE

The importance of quality of life is emphasized by patient-centred care when evaluating alternative therapies for cancer treatment. This approach mainly prioritizes the alignment of treatment decisions with the preferences of patients' values and overall health of patients rather than only focusing on the clinical outcome. Different cancer treatment methods will impact the quality of life in various ways. Research has shown that cervical cancer patients who had undergone surgery alone reported having a higher quality of life with improved physical, emotional and social functioning when compared to those who had received RT or combined therapy (Sorokin et al., 2024). These findings showed the necessity for a personalized treatment method to focus on patients' wellbeing over a one-size-fits-all approach. Patient-reported outcomes (PROs) are pivotal in assessing quality of life and shaping treatment decisions. PROs help patients have firsthand experiences and preferences, thus providing various information regarding clinician insights. Utilizing PROs can help improve patient engagement, help foster open communication and help increase patient satisfaction with care. This will lead to improved health outcomes for the cancer patient (Wang & Bellows, 2018). Integrative medicine will combine conventional and alternative therapy to align with the principles of patient-centred care. Integrative medicine mainly emphasizes holistic healing and respects the preferences of individuals making this approach more valuable for addressing quality-of-life considerations (George, 2015). Despite limited empirical support for its efficacy, its growing acceptance highlights patients' demand for more personalized care options.

While quality-of-life considerations are vital, some patients may prioritize survival over quality of life, presenting a complex dynamic in treatment decisions. Balancing these priorities requires nuanced understanding and shared decision-making to ensure effective patient-centred care.

GLOBAL ACCESSIBILITY AND COST-EFFECTIVENESS OF ALTERNATIVE CANCER TREATMENTS

Cost Comparison of Proton Therapy

Proton therapy is a highly advanced radiation modality that precisely targets tumours while minimizing damage to surrounding healthy tissues. However, its high cost presents a significant barrier to widespread adoption. A single proton therapy session can range from $30,000 to $50,000, making it substantially more expensive than traditional RTs, which typically cost between $8,000 and $20,000 per course of treatment. As a result, proton therapy remains largely restricted to high-income countries and major cancer centres with specialized facilities (Cohen et al., 2022). Expanding insurance coverage and developing cost-reduction strategies are crucial for improving access to this innovative treatment.

Focused Ultrasound Accessibility

FUS is an emerging non-invasive technology used in cancer treatment, particularly for prostate, liver and pancreatic cancers. Despite its benefits, accessibility remains limited due to high equipment costs and the need for specialized training. The cost of acquiring and maintaining FUS technology can exceed $500,000, restricting its use primarily to research institutions and leading cancer hospitals. Additionally, the expertise required for FUS procedures further limits its adoption in low-resource settings. Expanding training programmes and investing in cost-effective models of FUS implementation could enhance its availability worldwide (Panzone et al., 2022).

Cost-Effectiveness of Radiofrequency Ablation

RF ablation is a widely used, minimally invasive technique for treating tumours in the liver, lungs and kidneys. Compared to surgical resection, RF ablation offers a cost-effective alternative with shorter hospital stays and lower procedural costs. The average cost of RF ablation ranges from $5,000 to $10,000 per procedure, depending on tumour size and location. Additionally, RF ablation's outpatient nature reduces indirect costs related to hospitalization and post-surgical care. Studies have shown that RF ablation can achieve comparable long-term survival rates to surgery in selected patient populations, making it a valuable option for both high- and low-income healthcare settings (Gallego Vilar et al., 2010).

Global Disparities in Access to Alternative Modalities

Access to alternative cancer treatments varies significantly across different regions. While developed countries invest in advanced therapies such as proton therapy and HIFU, low- and middle-income nations often face barriers due to economic constraints, inadequate infrastructure and limited healthcare resources. In high-income countries like the United States, Japan and Germany, patients have access to cutting-edge technologies, clinical trials and multidisciplinary treatment teams. Conversely, in many developing nations, cancer patients primarily rely on conventional therapies such as chemotherapy and surgery due to financial limitations and lack of specialized equipment.

Efforts to bridge this gap include international collaborations, government subsidies and technology-sharing initiatives. For example, partnerships between healthcare institutions in high-income and low-income countries have facilitated knowledge transfer and improved access to novel therapies. Additionally, non-profit organizations and global health agencies continue to advocate for the equitable distribution of cancer treatment resources (Schippers & Lomax, 2011).

Global Optimization Efforts and Strategies

Global optimization in healthcare, particularly in cancer treatment, is increasingly reliant on international collaborations, harmonization of clinical guidelines and technology transfer. These strategies aim to enhance treatment modalities and improve patient outcomes across diverse healthcare systems.

INTERNATIONAL COLLABORATIONS AND RESEARCH NETWORKS

Multinational research consortia play a crucial role in advancing cancer research and treatment by fostering partnerships between institutions in high-income countries and those in low- and middle-income countries. One notable example is the Breast Health Global Initiative (BHGI), which collaborates with low- and middle-income countries to improve breast cancer care through resource-stratified guidelines (Anderson et al., 2006). Another initiative, the International Cancer Genome Consortium (ICGC), facilitates the global sharing of genomic data, enabling researchers to study cancer genetics across different populations (Boutros et al., 2014).

Shared research data from such collaborations contribute to a deeper understanding of cancer genomics and treatment efficacy. Additionally, international clinical trials involving diverse patient populations improve the generalizability of findings and support the optimization of treatment modalities (Al-Sukhun et al., 2017). These collaborations bridge the gap in knowledge and access, ultimately fostering equitable healthcare advancements.

Harmonization of Clinical Guidelines

Efforts to create international consensus guidelines are essential for integrating alternative treatment modalities with conventional therapies. Organizations such as the National Comprehensive Cancer Network (NCCN) and the World Health Organization (WHO) work toward standardizing treatment protocols to ensure their applicability across various healthcare settings (Al-Sukhun et al., 2017).

Standardized clinical guidelines provide a framework for evidence-based practice, improving the quality of care regardless of economic and technological disparities. Resource-stratified guidelines, such as those developed by the BHGI and WHO, help healthcare providers in low- and middle-income countries optimize resource allocation and implement cost-effective cancer treatment strategies (Anderson et al., 2006). These harmonized guidelines promote equity in care delivery by ensuring that essential cancer treatments are accessible across different healthcare systems.

Technology Transfer and Capacity Building

Transferring advanced treatment technologies to resource-limited settings is a critical component of global optimization. HIFU, RF ablation and proton therapy are among the technologies being introduced through international initiatives. Programmes such as the International Atomic Energy Agency's (IAEA) Rays of Hope initiative focus on enhancing RT capabilities in low- and middle-income countries. Capacity-building strategies include specialized training programmes for local healthcare professionals, enabling them to utilize these advanced technologies effectively. Additionally, funding partnerships between governments, non-profit organizations and private-sector entities support infrastructure development and technology acquisition. These initiatives collectively contribute to reducing disparities in cancer care and improving global health outcomes.

INTERNATIONAL COLLABORATIONS AND RESEARCH NETWORKS

Multinational research consortia and partnerships play a critical role in advancing global healthcare optimization. Organizations such as the IARC and the Global Alliance for Genomics and Health (GA4GH) foster collaboration between high-income countries and institutions in low- and middle-income regions (Chinnathambi, 2024). For example, the African Organization for Research and Training in Cancer (AORTIC) partners with major cancer centres in Europe and North America to enhance oncology research and clinical trials in Africa (Vij, 2024). Shared research data and multinational clinical trials contribute to optimizing treatment modalities by ensuring broader genetic and environmental representation, leading to more effective and inclusive therapeutic strategies (Oyediran et al., 2024). These collaborations enable knowledge exchange, technology transfer and improved patient outcomes across diverse healthcare settings (Berros et al., 2023).

Harmonization of Clinical Guidelines

Efforts to create international consensus guidelines for integrating alternative modalities with conventional treatments are gaining momentum. The WHO and the European Society for Medical Oncology (ESMO) have initiated global frameworks to standardize integrative oncology approaches (Chinnathambi, 2024). A notable example is the collaboration between the American Society of Clinical Oncology (ASCO) and global partners to develop guidelines for complementary therapies such as acupuncture and herbal medicine in cancer care (Vij, 2024). Standardized protocols facilitate the adaptation of treatment strategies to various healthcare systems, ensuring that patients in different regions receive consistent and evidence-based care. Such harmonization minimizes disparities in treatment accessibility and quality while promoting interdisciplinary research on the efficacy and safety of alternative treatments (Berros et al., 2023).

Technology Transfer and Capacity Building

Programmes focused on transferring advanced treatment technologies, such as HIFU, RF ablation and proton therapy, to resource-limited settings are vital for global healthcare optimization. Initiatives like the Global Health Innovative Technology Fund (GHIT) and Access to Advanced Health Institute (AAHI) support the deployment of cutting-edge medical technologies in underserved regions (Chinnathambi, 2024). Training programmes, such as the IAEA oncology fellowship for RT specialists, enhance the local capacity to implement sophisticated treatment options (Vij, 2024). International funding partnerships, including public–private collaborations, further drive these advancements by providing financial resources and technical expertise. Organizations such as the WHO and the Gates Foundation play a crucial role in boosting healthcare infrastructure, ensuring that technological advancements reach those in need (Berros et al., 2023).

By strengthening international collaborations, standardizing clinical guidelines and facilitating technology transfer, the global healthcare community can optimize treatment strategies and improve patient outcomes worldwide.

CASE STUDIES

Exploring alternative modalities in cancer treatment has yielded promising case studies demonstrating successful patient outcomes. These examples highlight the potential of integrating complementary therapies with conventional treatments, showcasing improved quality of life and, in some cases, complete remission.

Histotripsy is an emerging technology utilizing HIFU to disrupt cancerous tissues through controlled cavitation. This method spares surrounding healthy tissues and offers a non-invasive approach to cancer treatment. Clinical applications have shown effective outcomes in various cancers, including liver and pancreatic cancers, with ongoing research indicating its potential to revolutionize cancer care (Parashar et al., 2024). In one case, a patient with recurrent liver cancer experienced complete tumour ablation using histotripsy, demonstrating its potential to provide effective treatment without the side effects of traditional therapies. These findings underscore the need for further clinical trials to validate histotripsy's efficacy as a mainstream cancer treatment.

A comprehensive study involving 232 cancer patients revealed that 66.4% found CAM compelling when combined with conventional chemotherapy. Among these therapies, herbal interventions, mainly green tea and black seeds, were reported as beneficial by 31.5% of patients (Keramatikerman, 2020; Rasheed et al., 2020). For example, a gastric cancer patient achieved complete remission and has remained cancer-free for over 9 years after integrating a herbal regimen with conventional treatments (Q & Q, 2015). This case highlights how herbal therapies can provide long-term benefits, especially when personalized to the patient's condition and used alongside conventional care.

Integrative oncology combines conventional and alternative modalities and has yielded promising outcomes. In a notable case of cervical cancer, a personalized treatment plan incorporating biological therapies and CAM was implemented based on the patient's genetic profile. This approach significantly improved treatment outcomes, emphasizing the importance of tailoring cancer therapies to individual patient characteristics (Chizenga & Abrahamse, 2021). Another successful case involved a pancreatic cancer patient who experienced extended survival and improved quality of life through a regimen that combined herbal medicine with chemotherapy. Such examples underline the potential of integrative approaches to enhance the effectiveness of standard treatments.

Nutritional support plays a critical role in improving treatment outcomes and patient wellbeing. A compelling case report described a metastatic breast cancer patient who underwent chemotherapy alongside a structured nutritional support programme. The patient achieved complete remission, with no evidence of recurrence, nearly 3 years post-treatment (Taxman et al., 2016). This case highlights the importance of addressing nutritional needs as part of a holistic cancer treatment strategy, particularly for patients undergoing aggressive therapies.

A remarkable long-term case of a colon cancer patient who integrated Ayurvedic practices with surgical interventions demonstrates the potential of traditional medicine to complement modern treatments. Diagnosed in 1995, the patient managed multiple recurrences of cancer over 24 years, maintaining a good quality of life and effectively treating uterine and renal cancers through this integrated approach (Bhatta, 2020). This case underscores the value of combining traditional and modern treatments to optimize patient outcomes.

While these case studies illustrate the effectiveness of alternative modalities, it is essential to consider the variability in patient responses. Further research is needed to establish standardized protocols for integrating these therapies into conventional cancer care. By combining evidence-based alternative treatments with conventional modalities, healthcare providers can offer personalized and holistic care, potentially improving outcomes for cancer patients.

ARTIFICIAL INTELLIGENCE TOOLS AIDING RADIATION THERAPY OMISSION DECISIONS

Artificial intelligence (AI) tools have become instrumental in personalizing cancer treatment plans, particularly in determining when RT can be safely omitted. IBM Watson for Oncology, for example, analyses clinical data, treatment guidelines and medical literature to assist oncologists in making evidence-based decisions. Despite its widespread adoption, some studies have raised concerns about Watson's recommendations, highlighting instances where suggested treatments were deemed unsafe or incorrect due to limitations in training data. RaySearch Laboratories' RayStation integrates machine learning algorithms to enhance treatment planning. By analysing patient-specific data, RayStation aids clinicians in optimizing treatment strategies, potentially identifying cases where RT omission is appropriate.

QUALITY-OF-LIFE BENEFITS IN PAEDIATRIC AND CENTRAL NERVOUS SYSTEM TUMORS

In paediatric oncology, especially concerning central nervous system (CNS) tumours, minimizing RT exposure is crucial due to the risk of long-term neurocognitive deficits. Studies have shown that proton beam radiotherapy (PBRT) results in significantly higher scores in neurocognitive outcomes, including IQ and memory, compared to conventional photon RT. This advantage is attributed to PBRT's precision in targeting tumours while sparing surrounding healthy tissue. Furthermore, the negative sequelae of RT in children are directly related to the volume of normal tissues exposed and the radiation dose received. Proton therapy, with its unique dose deposition pattern, reduces radiation exposure to normal brain tissue, thereby lowering the risk of cognitive dysfunction and enhancing health-related quality of life. The integration of AI tools in treatment planning and the adoption of advanced RT techniques like PBRT contribute to more personalized and effective cancer care, particularly in paediatric and CNS tumour cases, ultimately improving patient outcomes and quality of life.

REFERENCES

Allen, B. J., Bezak, E., & Marcu, L. G. (2013). Quo vadis radiotherapy? Technological advances and the rising problems in cancer management. *BioMed Research International, 2013*, 1–9. https://doi.org/10.1155/2013/749203

Al-Sukhun, S., De Lima Lopes, G., Gospodarowicz, M., Ginsburg, O., & Yu, P. P. (2017). Global health initiatives of the international oncology community. *American Society of Clinical Oncology Educational Book, 37*, 395–402. https://doi.org/10.1200/EDBK_100008

Anderson, B. O., Yip, C.-H., Ramsey, S. D., Bengoa, R., Braun, S., Fitch, M., Groot, M., Sancho-Garnier, H., Tsu, V. D., & Global Summit Health Care Systems and Public Policy Panel. (2006). Breast cancer in limited-resource countries: Health care systems and public policy. *Breast Journal, 12*(Suppl 1), S54–S69. https://doi.org/10.1111/j.1075-122X.2006.00203.x

Avedian, R. S., Bitton, R., Gold, G., Butts-Pauly, K., & Ghanouni, P. (2016). Is MR-guided high-intensity focused ultrasound a feasible treatment modality for desmoid tumors? *Clinical Orthopaedics & Related Research, 474*(3), 697–704. https://doi.org/10.1007/s11999-015-4364-0

Berros, N., El Mendili, F., Filaly, Y., & El Bouzekri El Idrissi, Y. (2023). Enhancing digital health services with big data analytics. *Big Data and Cognitive Computing, 7*(2), 64. https://doi.org/10.3390/bdcc7020064

Bhatta, P. (2020). Effectiveness of integrated approach on cancer care. *Europasian Journal of Medical Sciences, 2*(1), 94–98. https://doi.org/10.46405/ejms.v2i1.40

Blana, A., Rogenhofer, S., Ganzer, R., Lunz, J.-C., Schostak, M., Wieland, W. F., & Walter, B. (2008). Eight years' experience with high-intensity focused ultrasonography for treatment of localized prostate cancer. *Urology, 72*(6), 1329–1333; discussion 1333–1334. https://doi.org/10.1016/j.urology.2008.06.062

Boutros, P. C., Ewing, A. D., Ellrott, K., Norman, T. C., Dang, K. K., Hu, Y., Kellen, M. R., Suver, C., Bare, J. C., Stein, L. D., Spellman, P. T., Stolovitzky, G., Friend, S. H., Margolin, A. A., & Stuart, J. M. (2014). Global optimization of somatic variant identification in cancer genomes with a global community challenge. *Nature Genetics, 46*(4), 318–319. https://doi.org/10.1038/ng.2932

Chinnathambi, J. K. (2024). Harnessing data analytics and artificial intelligence in healthcare: A new dawn in patient care. *International Journal of Science & Technoledge*. https://doi.org/10.24940/theijst/2024/v12/i8/OJSST2408-001

Chizenga, E. P., & Abrahamse, H. (2021). Biological therapy with complementary and alternative medicine in innocuous integrative oncology: A case of cervical cancer. *Pharmaceutics, 13*(5), 626. https://doi.org/10.3390/pharmaceutics13050626

Chu, W. T. (1995). Ion beams for cancer treatment—A perspective. *Nuclear Instruments and Methods in Physics Research Section B: Beam Interactions with Materials and Atoms, 99*(1–4), 835–838. https://doi.org/10.1016/0168-583X(94)00616-4

Cohen, J., Alexander, G., & Mishra, M. V. (2022). Non-prostate genitourinary cancers. In T. D. Malouff & D. M. Trifiletti (Eds.), *Principles and Practice of Particle Therapy* (1st ed., pp. 411–423). Wiley. https://doi.org/10.1002/9781119707530.ch22

Gallego Vilar, D., José Povo Martin, I., Miralles Aguado, J., Garau Perelló, C., Bosquet Sanz, M., Gimeno Argente, V., Cifrián, M., García Vila, J., & Gallego Gómez, J. (2010). Radiofrequency ablation as an alternative treatment for organ confined renal tumor. *Actas Urológicas Españolas (English Edition), 34*(10), 860–865. https://doi.org/10.1016/S2173-5786(10)70214-6

Gazouli, I., Kyriazoglou, A., Kotsantis, I., Anastasiou, M., Pantazopoulos, A., Prevezanou, M., Chatzidakis, I., Kavourakis, G., Economopoulou, P., Kontogeorgakos, V., Papagelopoulos, P., & Psyrri, A. (2021). Systematic review of recurrent osteosarcoma systemic therapy. *Cancers, 13*(8), 1757. https://doi.org/10.3390/cancers13081757

George, M. (2015). Integrative medicine is integral to providing patient-centered care. *Annals of Allergy, Asthma & Immunology, 114*(4), 261–264. https://doi.org/10.1016/j.anai.2015.01.001

Hanna, N., Johnson, D., Temin, S., Baker, S., Brahmer, J., Ellis, P. M., Giaccone, G., Hesketh, P. J., Jaiyesimi, I., Leighl, N. B., Riely, G. J., Schiller, J. H., Schneider, B. J., Smith, T. J., Tashbar, J., Biermann, W. A., & Masters, G. (2017). Systemic therapy for stage IV non-small-cell lung cancer: American Society of Clinical Oncology clinical practice guideline update. *Journal of Clinical Oncology, 35*(30), 3484–3515. https://doi.org/10.1200/JCO.2017.74.6065

Keramatikerman, M. (2020). Efficacy of complementary and alternative therapies in cancer patients: A systematic review. *Biomedical Journal of Scientific & Technical Research, 29*(1). https://doi.org/10.26717/BJSTR.2020.29.004744

Kinsella, T. J (1981). New therapeutic strategies in radiation therapy. *245*(16), 1669. https://doi.org/10.1001/jama.1981.03310410047030

Michaels, A. Y., Keraliya, A. R., Tirumani, S. H., Shinagare, A. B., & Ramaiya, N. H. (2016). Systemic treatment in breast cancer: A primer for radiologists. *Insights into Imaging, 7*(1), 131–144. https://doi.org/10.1007/s13244-015-0447-4

Min, H.-Y., & Lee, H.-Y. (2022). Molecular targeted therapy for anticancer treatment. *Experimental & Molecular Medicine, 54*(10), 1670–1694. https://doi.org/10.1038/s12276-022-00864-3

Oyediran, M. O., Ojo, O. S., Raji, I. A., Adeniyi, A. E., & Aroba, O. J. (2024). An optimized support vector machine for lung cancer classification system. *Frontiers in Oncology, 14*, 1408199. https://doi.org/10.3389/fonc.2024.1408199

Panzone, J., Byler, T., Bratslavsky, G., & Goldberg, H. (2022). Applications of focused ultrasound in the treatment of genitourinary cancers. *Cancers, 14*(6), 1536. https://doi.org/10.3390/cancers14061536

Parashar, A. K., Tyagi, L. K., & Arora, V. (2024). Histotripsy: A promising modality for cancer treatment. *Current Cancer Therapy Reviews, 21*. https://doi.org/10.2174/0115733947330950240906075443

Q, Wei-Li, & Q, Si-Qi. (2015). Three cases of successful anticancer therapeutic regimens. *Journal of Medical Diagnostic Methods, 04*(04). https://doi.org/10.4172/2168- 9784.1000183

Rasheed, Z., Al-Rashidy, M., Al-Raqibah, A., Al-Moqbel, A., Al-Bakri, A., Al-Harbi, A., Rasheed, N., & Al Abdulmonem, W. (2020). Experience of cancer patients for the usage of complementary and alternative medicine therapy. *Open Access Macedonian Journal of Medical Sciences, 8*(E), 521–527. https://doi.org/10.3889/oamjms.2020.5012

Schippers, J. M., & Lomax, A. J. (2011). Emerging technologies in proton therapy. *Acta Oncologica, 50*(6), 838–850. https://doi.org/10.3109/0284186X.2011.582513

Shukla, A., & Bansal, V. (2015). Role of reradiation in head and neck cancer from limits to option. *Asian Journal of Oncology, 01*(01), 011–020. https://doi.org/10.4103/2454-6798.165084

Sorokin, P., Kulikova, S., Nikiforchin, A., & Ulrikh, E. (2024). Impact of various treatment modalities on long-term quality of life in cervical cancer survivors. *Cureus*. https://doi.org/10.7759/cureus.68642

Taxman, E. T., Conlon, E. D., Speers, A., Dismuke, K. L., Heyman, T. S., & Taxman, T. L. (2016). Chemotherapy and functional medicine in a patient with metastatic breast cancer: A case report. *Integrative Medicine (Encinitas, Calif.), 15*(1), 27–32.

Tiefenbacher, A., & Pirker, R. (2018). Systemic treatment of advanced non-small cell lung cancer: Controversies and perspectives. *Memo—Magazine of European Medical Oncology, 11*(2), 112–115. https://doi.org/10.1007/s12254-018-0408-y

Van Houtte, P., Florian, C., Moretti, L., & Van Gestel, D. (2021). Radiotherapy: An alternative to surgery. In H. S. Park (Ed.), *Lung Cancer—Modern Multidisciplinary Management*. IntechOpen. https://doi.org/10.5772/intechopen.94486

Vij, R. (2024). Revolutionizing healthcare. In A. Kaur, C. Kaushal, Md. M. Hassan, & S. T. Aung, *Federated Deep Learning for Healthcare* (1st ed., pp. 17–30). CRC Press. https://doi.org/10.1201/9781032694870-2

Wang, M. C., & Bellows, J. (2018). Quality of life and patient-centered outcomes. In T. P. Daaleman & M. R. Helton (Eds.), *Chronic Illness Care* (pp. 95–107). Springer International Publishing. https://doi.org/10.1007/978-3-319-71812-5_8

Patient Selection Standards

Recognizing Potential NO-RT Candidates

Peeyush Shukla and Shrikant Khare

SELECTION CRITERIA—DETAILED CRITERIA FOR IDENTIFYING PATIENTS WHO MIGHT BENEFIT FROM NO-RT

Identification of patients who might benefit from no radiation therapy (NO-RT) mainly involves a comprehensive assessment of clinical and paraclinical criteria. This selection process ensures that patients receive personalized treatment and also avoids unnecessary radiation exposure. The detailed criteria based on the latest research for identification of the potential of NO-RT candidates are given in **Figure 5.1**. Nanograms are

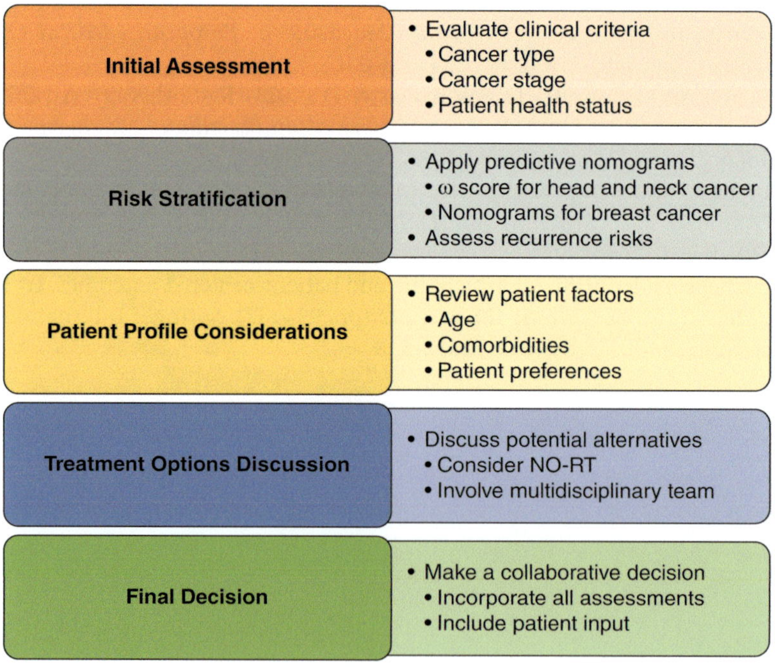

FIGURE 5.1 Identification of NO-RT candidates.

DOI: 10.1201/9781003529071-5

becoming more valuable in the prediction of outcomes in specific patient groups. For example, a nanogram that is developed for patients with pT1-T2N1 breast cancer post-mastectomy helps in evaluating the overall survival rates. Some studies showing that the lowest patients are classified by using nanograms have shown no significant overall survival rate improvement with postmastectomy radiotherapy. These groups of patients might safely not undergo radiation and can rely on an alternative therapeutic approach (Tang et al., 2020).

For head and neck cancer patients, the ω score nomogram helps in assessing the likelihood of cancer requirements against mortality risks. Patients with low ω scores indicate a minimal recurrence rate, and they may not benefit from intense treatments like radiotherapy. Identifying these types of patients can allow clinicians to focus on less aggressive but equally effective treatment (Vitzthum et al., 2020). In terms of rectal cancer, achieving a complete response for neoadjuvant radiochemotherapy can help eliminate the need for surgery and radiation. In adopting this approach there is a need for critical selection based on the stringent criteria for making sure of the oncological safety and reduction in the physical burden of patients (Marincaş et al., 2015). The tumour's histological features and the degree of peritoneal spread are taken into consideration when choosing patients for operations like cytoreductive surgery combined with hyperthermic intraperitoneal chemotherapy (HIPEC). The critical factors are favourable tumour histology and limited malignant spread. Patients who meet these criteria will have low recurrence rates and may even avoid radiation therapy (RT) without compromising any outcomes (Sammartino et al., 2015). Patient selection for NO-RT is very important and requires careful consideration of individual health, preferences and clinical data for comparisons. The decision to exclude RT must be made collaboratively with healthcare providers by discussing the potential benefits and risks with the patient. This personalized approach can ensure optimal care and also reduce unnecessary treatment. For a visual overview, please refer to **Figure 5.2**.

SUITABILITY INTERNATIONAL STANDARDS AND GUIDELINES

In today's complex healthcare environment, integrating established international standards is essential for enhancing the patient selection process for RT and alternative treatments. Adopting these standards ensures that clinicians follow evidence-based protocols and align their practices with global benchmarks, resulting in more consistent and effective treatment plans.

The American Society for Radiation Oncology (ASTRO) provides comprehensive guidelines that assist clinicians in evaluating a patient's overall health, medical history and treatment objectives. These guidelines help to ensure that RT is offered to those most likely to benefit, thereby reducing unnecessary exposure and maximizing therapeutic success. Similarly, the European Society for Radiotherapy and Oncology (ESTRO) emphasizes precision and safety in radiation delivery. Their recommendations focus on advanced technology and rigorous patient assessments to optimize treatment outcomes while minimizing risks.

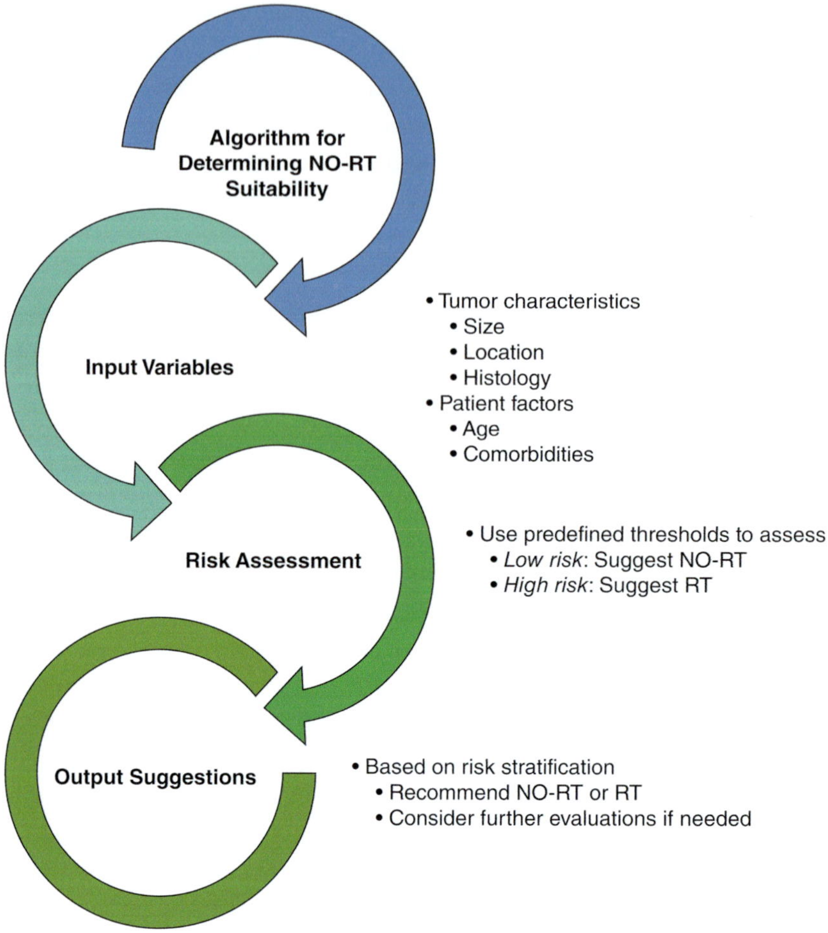

FIGURE 5.2 Algorithm for determining NO-RT.

The International Atomic Energy Agency (IAEA) contributes by establishing robust safety standards and best practices in RT. IAEA protocols serve as a framework to protect patients from potential adverse effects by promoting high levels of safety in both planning and treatment execution. Complementing these guidelines, the National Comprehensive Cancer Network (NCCN) offers clinical practice recommendations that support clinicians in making informed decisions about various cancer treatment options. The NCCN guidelines are particularly useful in identifying candidates for alternative therapies that do not involve radiation, based on a thorough evaluation of clinical evidence.

Moreover, the World Health Organization (WHO) advocates for the integration of evidence-based practices in healthcare. WHO recommendations encourage the adoption of internationally recognized protocols into local clinical settings, thereby enhancing the overall quality of patient care. This strategic alignment with global standards not only strengthens the credibility of the patient selection process but also facilitates meaningful comparisons of treatment outcomes across different regions.

Ultimately, the adoption of international standards fosters a systematic, transparent and scientifically sound approach to patient selection. By integrating guidelines from ASTRO, ESTRO, IAEA, NCCN and WHO, healthcare providers ensure that every decision is based on the latest evidence. This commitment to global best practices not only enhances clinical decision-making but also leads to improved patient outcomes and a higher standard of care.

By adhering to these international guidelines, healthcare systems promote consistency and encourage continuous improvement in clinical practices. The harmonization of local protocols with globally accepted standards empowers clinicians to make decisions that are both innovative and grounded in scientific rigor, ultimately leading to a safer, more effective treatment environment. This benefits all patients.

RISK STRATIFICATION—TOOLS AND TECHNIQUES FOR ASSESSING PATIENT RISK

One of the critical processes in healthcare that helps clinicians determine patient risk effectively is risk stratification. This can be particularly used in procedures like transcatheter aortic valve replacement (TAVR) and coronary interventions. With the help of various tools and techniques, healthcare providers can ensure the right procedures are performed at the right time. This section discusses methodologies and tools used in risk stratification, focusing on predictive models and their applications.

Some of the risk stratification tools are risk scores, predictive models and machine learning techniques. Risk scores are important for the evaluation of cardiovascular and non-cardiovascular predictors of patients that help clinicians make informed decisions about procedures like TAVR. These scores combine multiple variables such as age, comorbidities and hemodynamic parameters to predict outcomes, hence helping to enhance procedural safety and effectiveness (Singh & Vallabhajosyula, 2024). Predictive models like the Risk Stratification Index 3.0 use a broad dataset based on International Classification of Diseases, Tenth Edition (ICD-10) codes to estimate the likelihood of adverse events. Validation studies of this index have demonstrated an average area under the curve (AUC) of 0.76, showcasing its reliability in clinical applications (Greenwald et al., 2022). Machine learning methods have emerged as promising tools for risk stratification. These techniques include random forests and neural networks. This improves the predictive accuracy by analysing complex patterns in patient data. Studies comparing machine learning approaches to traditional logistic regression have shown similar predictive performances, reinforcing their utility in risk assessments (Greenwald et al., 2022).

The patient selection standards are mainly based on comorbidities and preferences. Effective risk stratification considers patient-specific factors such as comorbidities, coronary anatomy and personal preferences. These elements are vital for tailoring interventions, ensuring that treatments align with patient goals and medical needs (Farooq & Serruys, 2018). A systematic, two-step approach to patient selection involving initial broad stratification followed by detailed risk assessment can optimize resource utilization and improve clinical outcomes. This strategy facilitates the identification of high-risk patients while minimizing unnecessary interventions (Dom Dera, 2019).

While risk stratification tools can significantly improve patient selection for procedures, there are still some challenges remaining. Over-reliance on predictive models may overlook unique patient circumstances, leading to suboptimal care. Moreover, concerns about the ethical implications of denying care to high-risk patients based on algorithmic predictions highlight the need for judicious application of these tools (Glance et al., 2022). Risk stratification is indispensable in modern healthcare, offering tools and techniques that improve decision-making and patient outcomes. However, achieving a balance between predictive accuracy and individualized care is essential to ensure ethical and effective healthcare delivery.

REAL-WORLD EXAMPLES OF SUCCESSFUL RISK STRATIFICATION

Risk stratification plays a crucial role in modern oncology by helping clinicians tailor treatments based on an individual's likelihood of disease progression, recurrence or treatment response. By using predictive models, biomarkers and clinical criteria, doctors can minimize unnecessary treatments, reduce side effects and improve patient outcomes. Discussed next are several real-world examples where risk stratification has significantly influenced treatment decisions.

Breast Cancer Risk Stratification

Breast cancer treatment decisions often rely on risk assessment tools that predict the need for additional therapies. A study focusing on patients with pT1-T2N1 breast cancer used a validated nanogram to evaluate the benefits of postmastectomy RT. The findings indicated that some patients did not experience a significant improvement in overall survival with RT, leading to the successful identification of individuals who could avoid unnecessary radiation exposure (Tang et al., 2020). This form of risk stratification prevented overtreatment while maintaining excellent oncologic outcomes. Instead of a one-size-fits-all approach, treatment was tailored based on tumour characteristics, optimizing patient care and quality of life. In addition to the nanogram-based criteria described by Tang et al. (2020), these parameters are in accordance with the latest recommendations from the NCCN, which emphasize a risk-adapted approach to minimize overtreatment.

Head and Neck Cancer Nomogram

For head and neck cancer, treatment decisions typically include surgery, radiation or chemotherapy, but not all patients require aggressive therapies. A study utilizing the ω score nomogram demonstrated how this tool could effectively identify individuals at low risk of recurrence who might not benefit from high-intensity treatments like RT. Patients classified with low ω scores were successfully managed with less intensive therapies, reducing unnecessary radiation exposure and its associated toxicities (Vitzthum et al., 2020). This case highlights the role of precision medicine in minimizing overtreatment while still ensuring adequate disease control. The ω score nomogram's application aligns with the guidelines set forth by ESTRO, which advocate for precision medicine in head and neck cancer management, further reinforcing the tool's clinical utility.

Risk Stratification in Rectal Cancer and Neoadjuvant Therapy

In rectal cancer, neoadjuvant chemoradiotherapy (CRT) is often used before surgery to shrink tumours and improve surgical outcomes. However, a clinical trial showed that patients who achieved a complete response to neoadjuvant CRT could be selected for surgery alone without additional RT. This strategy significantly reduced the overall treatment burden for eligible patients and improved their quality of life by sparing them the potential side effects of further radiation (Marincaş et al., 2015). By implementing strict selection criteria, clinicians were able to personalize treatment, ensuring that only those who truly needed additional RT received it.

Cytoreductive Surgery and Hyperthermic Intraperitoneal Chemotherapy

For patients with peritoneal carcinomatosis, an advanced form of cancer that spreads within the abdominal cavity, risk stratification has played a vital role in guiding treatment. Patients with favourable tumour histology were identified through predictive models as ideal candidates for cytoreductive surgery combined with hyperthermic intraperitoneal chemotherapy (HIPEC). This tailored approach helped reduce recurrence rates, improve survival and, in some cases, allow patients to avoid RT altogether (Sammartino et al., 2015). The ability to stratify patients based on tumour biology and response to therapy has been instrumental in optimizing outcomes while minimizing unnecessary interventions.

These real-world examples demonstrate how risk stratification enhances personalized cancer treatment, allowing clinicians to avoid overtreatment, reduce unnecessary side effects and improve patient quality of life. The use of predictive models, genetic profiling and clinical decision tools continues to shape the future of oncology, ensuring that each patient receives the most effective, tailored therapy for their specific condition. As research progresses, the integration of artificial intelligence, big data and machine learning will further refine these risk assessment methods, ultimately leading to better outcomes and more efficient use of healthcare resources.

PATIENT PROFILES—SPECIFIC PATIENT GROUPS IDEAL FOR NO-RT

The ideal candidate for NO-RT consists of a specific group of patients who present unique challenges and need special management strategies in pre-operative care. By addressing their needs, NO-RT can be used as an alternative therapy for RT with optimized results and reduced risks.

Elderly patients have multiple comorbidities that increase the risks associated with surgical procedures. Age-related physiological changes, polypharmacy and reduced physiological reserve necessitate a thorough assessment of their medical status before considering surgical interventions. For these patients, NO-RT provides an opportunity to avoid the complications frequently associated with anaesthesia and invasive surgeries. Personalized approaches that focus on comorbidity management and functional status monitoring have proven effective in reducing perioperative risks (Prasad, 2022).

Pregnant patients who undergo non-obstetric surgeries represent another critical group for NO-RT. Surgical interventions during pregnancy may cause potential risks to both the mother and foetus, particularly during the first and third trimesters. The application of

NO-RT in such conditions provides an alternative to reduce these risks and also ensures effective management of the underlying conditions of patients. Multidisciplinary collaboration between obstetricians, anaesthesiologists and surgeons is essential to optimize outcomes and prioritize maternal and fetal safety (Prasad & May, 2019). Obese patients are at an increased risk for postoperative complications like infections, delayed wound healing and extended recovery times. These risks are increased by obesity-related comorbidities like sleep apnoea and cardiovascular issues. NO-RT serves as a beneficial approach for managing conditions within this patient group. This mainly focuses on pre-operative interventions like modifications in lifestyle and management of weight to improve overall health. This strategy reduces dependency on surgical solutions and encourages long-term wellness (Prasad, 2022).

Immunocompromised patients are those undergoing chemotherapy, organ transplant recipients or individuals with autoimmune disorders. They face an increased risk of infections and other complications post-surgery. Hospital environments are critical for recovery and may expose these patients to pathogens, and this increases their vulnerability. NO-RT can reduce hospital exposure while effectively addressing the medical needs of patients. The optimization of immune function and implementation of close monitoring protocols can help in improved outcomes for this group (Prasad & May, 2019).

For patients with chronic low back pain who do not respond to primary care treatments, NO-RT can serve as an effective alternative to surgery. Predictive models show that individuals with high disability levels and significant psychosocial complaints frequently show suboptimal responses to surgical interventions. However, NO-RT provides a non-invasive approach to alleviating pain and improving quality of life without the risks inherent in surgical procedures (Van Hooff et al., 2018).

Individuals with non-malignant conditions such as musculoskeletal disorders are often suitable candidates for NO-RT. The treatment not only reduces the symptoms but also improves their quality of life. This modality reduces the need for surgical interventions and their associated risks, positioning NO-RT as a practical choice for managing chronic, non-malignant ailments (Nardone et al., 2022).

Patients with chronic diseases like type 2 diabetes can benefit significantly from NO-RT. Personalized management strategies that consider their specific profiles have been shown to improve the efficacy of treatment, improve satisfaction and reduce the risks associated with surgical care. Integrating personalized care plans within NO-RT frameworks helps in achieving better outcomes for this patient group (Elissen et al., 2016).

While NO-RT offers advantages for these patient groups, it may not be appropriate for individuals requiring immediate surgical intervention or acute care. Balancing the risks and benefits and employing a patient-centred approach is key to identifying ideal candidates and optimizing treatment pathways.

MULTIDISCIPLINARY EVALUATION—ROLE OF THE MULTIDISCIPLINARY TEAM IN SELECTING NO-RT CANDIDATES

The multidisciplinary team (MDT) plays an important role in the identification of suitable candidates for NO-RT in cancer management. The integration of expertise from various medical disciplines helps in patient care, allows for personalized treatment plans and reduces any unnecessary interventions. MDTs are necessary for the evaluation of the eligibility of patients for NO-RT by a complete assessment of clinical and personal factors. These teams can help in evaluating the stage of the disease, comorbidities and overall patient health and also help in recommending appropriate treatment options. For example, the assessment of MDTs has been shown to improve the decision-making process significantly. This can provide a personalized recommendation based on clinical and patient-centred data (Martini et al., 2022). MDT discussions often result in changes to initial treatment strategies and resolve disagreements through collaborative efforts. This can be seen in colorectal cancer management, where MDT deliberations have been associated with improved treatment outcomes and minimized variations in care (Anghelone et al., 2022; Elsaadi & Jahany, 2023).

MDTs operate in a collaborative framework that involves oncologists, surgeons, radiologists and other specialists. This enables a holistic review of patient conditions and available treatment modalities (Ichikawa et al., 2022). This approach ensures that decisions are informed by a multidisciplinary perspective, thus helping in the precision and relevance of treatment recommendations. Including the preferences of patients in the decision-making process is an important feature of MDTs. This patient-centred approach ensures that the treatment plan will align with the individual values and clinical evidence. This helps in fostering trust and adherence to therapy. MDT recommendations can help in reducing the likelihood of unnecessary radiation therapy. This shows the importance of shared decision-making frameworks (Ichikawa et al., 2022). One of the important responsibilities of MDTs is to analyse and assess the alternatives to RT. This includes assessing surgery, systemic therapies or other non-invasive options. MDT evaluations have played a significant role in pancreatic cancer management, where treatment allocation often varies. This shows the need for consistency in MDT recommendations to ensure optimal patient outcomes (Kirkegård et al., 2019; Milligan et al., 2022). In metastatic renal cell carcinoma, MDT discussions have been related to improved survival rates. This further validates the efficacy of a multidisciplinary approach to care planning (Zeng et al., 2023).

While MDTs significantly improve the decision-making processes, there are still some challenges that persist. Disagreements in treatment recommendations and variability in protocol implementation show the need for standardized practices. Additionally, improving data collection and reporting during MDT evaluations can help address gaps and ensure consistent care delivery. The MDT's collaborative framework is integral to the selection of NO-RT candidates, ensuring patient-centred and evidence-based care. By using diverse expertise and prioritizing shared decision-making, MDTs contribute to improved patient outcomes and satisfaction. However, continued efforts to refine MDT processes and overcome existing challenges are necessary to optimize their impact on cancer management fully.

ETHICAL CONSIDERATIONS—ADDRESSING THE ETHICAL IMPLICATIONS OF WITHHOLDING RADIATION THERAPY

The ethical implications of withholding RT are multifaceted, requiring a careful balance of fundamental principles such as beneficence, non-maleficence, autonomy and justice. International ethical standards like those outlined by the WHO (2019) and the International Agency for Research on Cancer (IARC, 2020). This emphasizes that these principles must guide clinical decisions when determining the appropriateness of withholding RT.

Beneficence and non-maleficence lie at the core of this ethical debate. Beneficence obligates clinicians to act in the best interest of the patient by providing treatments that offer substantial clinical benefits, while non-maleficence demands that any intervention avoid causing unnecessary harm. For instance, in managing orbital rhabdomyosarcoma, North American protocols often include up-front RT to reduce recurrence rates, whereas European strategies may favour withholding RT to mitigate long-term adverse effects such as radiation-induced secondary malignancies (Farnia et al., 2015; Schiappacasse, 2021). These contrasting approaches highlight the ongoing ethical balancing act between maximizing therapeutic benefits and minimizing potential harm—a balance also underscored by international ethical guidelines (Bochud et al., 2020).

Patient autonomy further requires that healthcare providers actively involve patients in treatment decisions through the process of informed consent. Global ethical standards insist that patients fully understand the potential benefits and risks of RT so they can make choices that reflect their personal values (Braun et al., 2019). Yet ethical tensions may arise when patients do not fully comprehend the implications of withholding therapy, thereby complicating the shared decision-making process (Manalo, 2013; De Crevoisier et al., 2023).

In resource-limited settings, ethical frameworks are particularly critical in guiding the allocation of scarce RT resources. Decisions here often involve prioritizing patients based on factors such as disease curability and the likelihood of achieving significant health outcomes (DeBoer et al., 2024). Moreover, effective communication remains vital in addressing these ethical complexities. In palliative care scenarios, for example, the decision to withhold RT may align with a patient's care goals, yet simultaneously generate moral distress among clinicians who struggle with the potential implications of such choices (Yerramilli et al., 2019).

By integrating international ethical standards with local clinical practices, clinicians can ensure that decisions regarding withholding RT are ethically justifiable. This alignment not only reinforces the principles of beneficence, non-maleficence and autonomy but also supports transparent, patient-centred care consistent with global ethical frameworks.

LUMINA TRIAL

The LUMINA trial and real-world data from Denmark provide valuable insights into the omission of RT in select breast cancer patients. However, both have limitations that must be considered when applying their findings to broader clinical practice.

Limitations of the LUMINA Trial

The LUMINA trial was a prospective study evaluating the omission of RT in women aged ≥55 years with low-risk luminal A breast cancer who underwent breast-conserving surgery and received endocrine therapy. While the 5-year local recurrence rate was low (2.3%), several limitations affect the generalizability of the results:

- **Age Restriction**: The trial included only women aged 55 and older, excluding younger patients who may have different tumour biology and higher recurrence risks. This age limitation restricts the applicability of the findings to a younger demographic.
- **Highly Selective Cohort**: Participants had to meet stringent criteria, including tumour size ≤2 cm, grade 1–2, oestrogen receptor (ER) ≥1%, progesterone receptor (PR) >20%, HER2-negative and Ki-67 ≤13.25%. Such strict inclusion criteria may not reflect the broader population of breast cancer patients (Offersen et al., 2022).
- **Short Follow-Up Duration**: With a median follow-up of 5 years, the study may not capture late recurrences, which are particularly relevant in hormone receptor-positive breast cancer.

These limitations suggest that while the LUMINA trial supports RT omission in a specific subset of patients, caution should be exercised before extending these findings to younger or higher-risk individuals.

REAL-WORLD DATA FROM DENMARK

Denmark's healthcare system has implemented nationwide protocols for breast cancer treatment, providing real-world data on RT practices. The Danish Breast Cancer Group (DBCG) conducted a randomized phase 3 trial comparing partial breast irradiation (PBI) to whole breast irradiation (WBI) in early breast cancer patients. The study found that PBI was non-inferior to WBI regarding breast induration, with similar recurrence rates over a median follow-up of 7.6 years. Building on these findings, the DBCG initiated the NATURAL trial (NCT03646955) to evaluate the omission of RT in patients meeting specific low-risk criteria. This ongoing study aims to provide further evidence on the safety and efficacy of omitting RT in carefully selected patients (Offersen et al., 2022). These real-world initiatives highlight the importance of individualized treatment approaches and the potential for safely omitting RT in certain patient populations. However, the applicability of these findings depends on strict adherence to selection criteria and may not be generalizable to all clinical settings.

While both the LUMINA trial and Danish real-world data support the omission of RT in select low-risk breast cancer patients, limitations such as age restrictions, stringent inclusion criteria and short follow-up periods necessitate cautious interpretation. Further research with more diverse populations and longer follow-up is essential to validate these approaches and ensure their safe implementation in broader clinical practice.

CONCLUSION

In conclusion, patient selection for NO-RT represents a paradigm shift towards more personalized and targeted healthcare, emphasizing the judicious use of medical interventions to enhance patient outcomes while minimizing unnecessary treatments. This nuanced approach, underpinned by rigorous clinical and paraclinical criteria, leverages tools such as predictive nomograms, risk stratification indices and machine learning models to identify suitable candidates for NO-RT across diverse patient groups. The involvement of MDTs is pivotal in this process, ensuring that decisions are informed by a holistic evaluation of patient-specific factors, disease characteristics and treatment alternatives. By integrating diverse expertise and prioritizing patient preferences, MDTs facilitate shared decision-making, fostering trust and adherence to personalized care plans. The collaborative framework also addresses challenges related to variability in recommendations and ethical considerations, balancing the principles of beneficence, non-maleficence, autonomy and justice. Furthermore, NO-RT presents a compelling option for special populations such as the elderly, pregnant individuals, immunocompromised patients and those with chronic or non-malignant conditions. These groups often benefit from reduced exposure to the risks associated with traditional therapies, underscoring the importance of tailored treatment pathways that align with their unique needs and health goals.

It is important to recognize that clinical practices and guidelines for NO-RT can vary significantly across regions, influenced by differences in healthcare infrastructure, regulatory policies and resource availability. Incorporating international standards not only supports evidence-based clinical decision-making but also fosters dialogue aimed at harmonizing practices across borders, ultimately enhancing global patient care.

Despite its advantages, NO-RT necessitates ongoing refinement to address challenges in implementation, standardization and ethical decision-making. Future efforts should focus on enhancing predictive accuracy, improving MDT processes and fostering patient education to ensure informed and equitable care. NO-RT exemplifies a patient-centred approach that aligns clinical innovations with individualized care, marking a significant advancement in the quest for precision medicine. By prioritizing evidence-based practices and ethical responsibility, this strategy holds the potential to transform cancer care and improve the quality of life for diverse patient populations.

REFERENCES

Anghelone, A., Bensi, M., Barbaro, B., Calegari, M. A., Cina, C., Menghi, R., Lorenzon, L., Pozzo, C., Basso, M., Schietroma, F., Valente, G., Lococo, F., Ardito, F., Cellini, F., Caira, G., Trovato, G., D'Ugo, D., Giuliante, F., Tortora, G., & Salvatore, L. (2022). The impact of the multidisciplinary team (MDT) in the management of colorectal cancer (CRC). *Journal of Clinical Oncology, 40*(16_suppl), e13641. https://doi.org/10.1200/JCO.2022.40.16_suppl.e13641

Bochud, F., Cantone, M. C., Applegate, K., Coffey, M., Damilakis, J., Del Rosario Perez, M., Fahey, F., Jesudasan, M., Kurihara-Saio, C., Le Guen, B., Malone, J., Murphy, M., Reid, L., & Zölzer, F. (2020). Ethical aspects in the use of radiation in medicine: Update from ICRP Task Group 109. *Annals of the ICRP, 49*(1_suppl), 143–153. https://doi.org/10.1177/0146645320929630

Braun, T. L., Patel, V., Dao Jr, H., & Rosen, T. (2019). What are the ethical and legal considerations when your patient refuses the standard of care? *Dermatology Online Journal, 25*(8). https://doi.org/10.5070/D3258045125

DeBoer, R. J., Ho, A., Mutoniwase, E., Nguyen, C., Umutesi, G., Bigirimana, J. B., Nsabimana, N., Van Loon, K., Shulman, L. N., Triedman, S. A., Cubaka, V. K., & Shyirambere, C. (2024). Ethical dilemmas in prioritizing patients for scarce radiotherapy resources. *BMC Medical Ethics, 25*(1), 12. https://doi.org/10.1186/s12910-024-01005-3

De Crevoisier, R., Leseur, J., Bouvet, C., Huguet, F., Lagrange, J.-L., Haaser, T., Pasquier, D., Créhange, G., Supiot, S., Pommier, P., Roy, A., Berna, A., Blanchard, P., & Marcucci, L. (2023). Compréhension/acceptation de la radiothérapie: Un dilemme éthique résolu par une éthique de la considération et de la sollicitude. *Cancer/Radiothérapie, 27*(2), 115–125. https://doi.org/10.1016/j.canrad.2022.08.005

Dom Dera, J. (2019). Risk stratification: A two-step process for identifying your sickest patients. *Family Practice Management, 26*(3), 21–26.

Elissen, A. M., Hertroijs, D. F., Schaper, N. C., Vrijhoef, H. J., & Ruwaard, D. (2016). Profiling patients' healthcare needs to support integrated, person-centered models for long-term disease management (profile): Research design. *International Journal of Integrated Care, 16*(2), 1. https://doi.org/10.5334/ijic.2208

Elsaadi, N. J., & Jahany, M. O. A. (2023). An investigative analysis of the role of multidisciplinary teams in cancer management: Assessing advantages and obstacles. *The Scientific Journal of University of Benghazi, 36*(1). https://doi.org/10.37376/sjuob.v36i1.3940

Farnia, B., Majumder, M. A., & Paulino, A. C. (2015). Ethical analysis as a tool for addressing treatment controversies: Radiotherapy timing in children with orbital rhabdomyosarcoma as a case example. *Journal of the American College of Radiology, 12*(5), 484–490. https://doi.org/10.1016/j.jacr.2014.10.010

Farooq, V., & Serruys, P. W. (2018). Risk stratification and risk scores. In W. Wijns (Ed.), *ESC Cardio Med* (pp. 1371–1384). Oxford University Press. https://doi.org/10.1093/med/9780198784906.003.0335

Glance, L. G., Vutskits, L., & Davidson, A. (2022). Prediction algorithms: Is peer review enough? *Anesthesiology, 137*(6), 661–663. https://doi.org/10.1097/ALN.0000000000004421

Greenwald, S., Chamoun, G. F., Chamoun, N. G., Clain, D., Hong, Z., Jordan, R., Manberg, P. J., Maheshwari, K., & Sessler, D. I. (2022). Risk stratification index 3.0, a broad set of models for predicting adverse events during and after hospital admission. *Anesthesiology, 137*(6), 673–686. https://doi.org/10.1097/ALN.0000000000004380

Ichikawa, M., Uematsu, K., Yano, N., Yamada, M., Ono, T., Kawashiro, S., Akamatsu, H., Hagiwara, Y., Sato, H., & Nemoto, K. (2022). Implementation rate and effects of multidisciplinary team meetings on decision making about radiotherapy: An observational study at a single Japanese institution. *BMC Medical Informatics and Decision Making, 22*(1), 111. https://doi.org/10.1186/s12911-022-01849-y

International Agency for Research on Cancer. (2020). *Promoting ethical and professional conduct*. International Agency for Research on Cancer. https://www.iarc.who.int/about-iarc-who-ethics/

Kirkegård, J., Aahlin, E. K., Al-Saiddi, M., Bratlie, S. O., Coolsen, M., De Haas, R. J., Den Dulk, M., Fristrup, C., Harrison, E. M., Mortensen, M. B., Nijkamp, M. W., Persson, J., Søreide, J. A., Wigmore, S. J., Wik, T., & Mortensen, F. V. (2019). Multicentre study of multidisciplinary team assessment of pancreatic cancer resectability and treatment allocation. *British Journal of Surgery, 106*(6), 756–764. https://doi.org/10.1002/bjs.11093

Manalo, M. F. C. (2013). End-of-life decisions about withholding or withdrawing therapy: Medical, ethical, and religio-cultural considerations. *Palliative Care: Research and Treatment, 7*, 1–5. https://doi.org/10.4137/PCRT.S10796

Marincaş, A. M., Prunoiu, V. M., Brătucu, E., Cirimbei, C., Ionescu, S., Buzatu, R., & Straja, N. D. (2015). Clinical and paraclinical criteria of patient selection for the non- operative treatment in completely responsive rectal cancer (after neoadjuvant radiochemotherapy). *Chirurgia (Bucharest, Romania: 1990), 110*(4), 351–355.

Martini, A., Fallara, G., Pellegrino, A. A., Nocera, L., Larcher, A., Raggi, D., Campi, R., Ploussard, G., Malavaud, B., Montorsi, F., Pal, S. K., Spiess, P. E., Choueiri, T. K., Necchi, A., & Capitanio, U. (2022). Multidisciplinary team referral at diagnosis for patients with non-metastatic renal cell carcinoma. *Urologic Oncology: Seminars and Original Investigations, 40*(8), 384.e9–384.e14. https://doi.org/10.1016/j.urolonc.2022.05.004

Milligan, M. G., Lennes, I. T., Hawari, S., Khandekar, M. J., Colson, Y., Shepard, J.-A. O., Frank, A., Sequist, L. V., Willers, H., & Keane, F. K. (2022). Incidence of radiation therapy among patients enrolled in a multidisciplinary pulmonary nodule and lung cancer screening clinic. *JAMA Network Open*, *5*(3), e224840. https://doi.org/10.1001/jamanetworkopen.2022.4840

Nardone, V., D'Ippolito, E., Grassi, R., Sangiovanni, A., Gagliardi, F., De Marco, G., Menditti, V. S., D'Ambrosio, L., Cioce, F., Boldrini, L., Salvestrini, V., Greco, C., Desideri, I., De Felice, F., D'Onofrio, I., Grassi, R., Reginelli, A., & Cappabianca, S. (2022). Non-oncological radiotherapy: A review of modern approaches. *Journal of Personalized Medicine*, *12*(10), 1677. https://doi.org/10.3390/jpm12101677

Offersen, B. V., Alsner, J., Nielsen, H. M., Jakobsen, E. H., Nielsen, M. H., Stenbygaard, L., Pedersen, A. N., Thomsen, M. S., Yates, E., Berg, M., Lorenzen, E. L., Jensen, I., Josipovic, M., Jensen, M.-B., Overgaard, J., & on behalf of the Danish Breast Cancer Group Radiotherapy Committee. (2022). Partial breast irradiation versus whole breast irradiation for early breast cancer patients in a randomized phase III trial: The Danish Breast Cancer Group partial breast irradiation trial. *Journal of Clinical Oncology*, *40*(36), 4189–4197. https://doi.org/10.1200/JCO.22.00451

Prasad, S. (2022). Challenging patient groups. *Surgery (Oxford)*, *40*(12), 784–789. https://doi.org/10.1016/j.mpsur.2022.10.020

Prasad, S., & May, H. (2019). Challenging patient groups. *Surgery (Oxford)*, *37*(12), 695–699. https://doi.org/10.1016/j.mpsur.2019.10.009

Sammartino, P., Accarpio, F., Sollazzo, B. M., Impagnatiello, A., Cornali, T., & Biacchi, D. (2015). Patient selection for treatment. In A. Di Giorgio & E. Pinto (Eds.), *Treatment of Peritoneal Surface Malignancies* (pp. 195–205). Springer Milan. https://doi.org/10.1007/978-88-470-5711-1_13

Schiappacasse, G. V. (2021). Ethical considerations in chemotherapy and vaccines in cancer patients in times of the COVID-19 pandemic. *Current Oncology*, *28*(3), 2007–2013. https://doi.org/10.3390/curroncol28030186

Singh, S., & Vallabhajosyula, P. (2024). Risk Scores (Risk Stratification). In P. W. Serruys, A. Cribier, H. Eltchaninoff, E. Grube, R. Makkar, Y. Onuma, J. G. Webb & M. B. Leon, *Transcatheter Aortic Valve Implantation* (2nd ed., pp. 50–55). CRC Press. https://doi.org/10.1201/9781003384779-6

Tang, Y., Zhang, Y.-J., Zhang, N., Shi, M., Wen, G., Cheng, J., Wang, H.-M., Liu, M., Wang, X.-H., Guo, Q.-S., Wu, H.-F., Ma, C.-Y., Jin, J., Liu, Y.-P., Song, Y.-W., Fang, H., Ren, H., Wang, S.-L., & Li, Y.-X. (2020). Nomogram predicting survival as a selection criterion for postmastectomy radiotherapy in patients with T1 to T2 breast cancer with 1 to 3 positive lymph nodes. *Cancer*, *126*(S16), 3857–3866. https://doi.org/10.1002/cncr.32963

Van Hooff, M. L., Van Dongen, J. M., Coupé, V. M., Spruit, M., Ostelo, R. W. J. G., & De Kleuver, M. (2018). Can patient-reported profiles avoid unnecessary referral to a spine surgeon? An observational study to further develop the Nijmegen decision tool for chronic low back pain. *PLoS One*, *13*(9), e0203518. https://doi.org/10.1371/journal.pone.0203518

Vitzthum, L. K., Park, H., Zakeri, K., Bryant, A. K., Feng, C., Shen, H., Cohen, E. E. W., Murphy, J. D., & Mell, L. K. (2020). Selection of head and neck cancer patients for intensive therapy. *International Journal of Radiation Oncology*Biology*Physics*, *106*(1), 157–166. https://doi.org/10.1016/j.ijrobp.2019.09.011

World Health Organization. (2022). *Ethics and medical radiological imaging: A policy brief for health professionals*. World Health Organization. https://doi.org/10.1016/j.clon.2020.03.006

Yerramilli, D., Parker, G., LeBaron, V., Krishnan, M., Hertan, L., Spektor, A., Shiloh, R., Skamene, S., & Balboni, T. (2019). Ethical issues in patients referred for palliative radiation therapy. *Annals of Palliative Medicine*, *8*(3), 231–239. https://doi.org/10.21037/apm.2019.06.02

Zeng, Y., Zhu, S., Wang, Z., Chen, J., Dai, J., Liu, Z., Sun, G., Liang, J., Zhang, X., Wang, Z., Zhao, J., Ni, Y., Yang, J., Wang, M., Wei, Q., Li, X., Chen, N., Li, Z., Wang, X., … Shen, P. (2023). Multidisciplinary team (MDT) discussion improves overall survival outcomes for metastatic renal cell carcinoma patients. *Journal of Multidisciplinary Healthcare*, *16*, 503–513. https://doi.org/10.2147/JMDH.S393457

CHAPTER 6

Clinical Determination

Handling Therapy Algorithms

Pooja Thakare and Gagandipsingh Bhamra

DECISION-MAKING FRAMEWORKS—DEVELOP AND EXPLAIN ALGORITHMS FOR DECIDING WHEN TO USE NO-RADIATION THERAPY

In oncology, the decision-making frameworks for no radiation therapy (NO-RT) play an important role in the optimization of health outcomes. This can help in reducing unnecessary treatment risks. These frameworks include structured algorithms, clinical evidence and patient-centred data for improving decision-making and minimizing subjective biases. The NOMS framework evaluates neurologic, oncologic, mechanical instability, and systemic disease (NOMS) factors for guiding the appropriateness of treatment options like radiation therapy (RT) or surgery (Bilsky & Azeem, 2007). In terms of NO-RT, this decision-making framework helps oncologists identify scenarios where systemic or mechanical factors will be more complex compared to the potential benefits of radiation. For example, patients with minimal systemic involvement or low oncologic burden may achieve better outcomes with non-radiation approaches. Clinical algorithms act as a tool for standardizing the decision-making and that helps in reducing cognitive biases and relies on intuition. These algorithms evaluate the patient-specific data for recommending evidence-based treatments that include NO-RT in some cases (Dennstädt et al., 2021). Algorithms in radiation oncology help in guiding the dose prescriptions but can be adapted for determining if the radiation may be avoided. By combining statistical models and the clinical trial results, these algorithms can help in decision-making with consideration of objective and patient-specific qualities.

Artificial intelligence (AI) systems like Adaptive Response Clinical Decision Support (ARCliDS) are transformative in clinical oncology. ARCliDS uses multi-omics data and helps in dynamically adjusting treatment recommendations for optimization of tumour control and reduction of side effects (Niraula et al., 2023). In terms of NO-RT, AI can help in predicting scenarios where alternative therapies or treatment methods like surgery or systemic therapies may be effective. These methods can provide comparable or superior outcomes without any risks related to radiation exposure. A

DOI: 10.1201/9781003529071-6

structured approach helps in evaluating the clinical trials and is essential for the adoption of NO-RT. The TARGIT-A trial has demonstrated benefit. This sets a precedent for exploring NO-RT options in some specific cases (Esserman et al., 2014). Assessing such trials in the adoption frameworks ensures that the innovations in the therapy are evidence based and aligned with the needs of the patient. Developing algorithms for NO-RT involved analysing key decision factors such as patient preferences, clinical evidence and risk–benefit ratios. These algorithms include genomic data and clinical data for the identification of patients who are most likely to benefit from avoiding RT (Lin, 2020). Structured algorithms improve decision-making by systematically assessing patient data and guiding oncologists towards optimal treatment strategies (Dennstädt et al., 2021; Ribi et al., 2022).

AI-driven adaptive systems like ARCliDS provide real-time decision support by predicting treatment outcomes using patient-specific data. These systems help in refining the recommendations dynamically and integrating new data as it becomes available to support personalized treatment plans (Niraula et al., 2023). In NO-RT these systems help oncologists with personalized interventions that align with evolving clinical evidence and patient needs. While structured algorithms and AI systems significantly improve the decision-making process, the complexity of oncology makes it necessary to find a balance between algorithmic objectivity and clinical judgment. Frameworks for NO-RT must integrate patient-centred approaches to address the nuanced requirements of individual cases. These decision-making tools aim to improve patient care by optimizing treatment outcomes, reducing unnecessary interventions and supporting evidence-based clinical decisions.

DECISION-MAKING MODELS DERIVED FROM MAJOR CLINICAL TRIALS

Major clinical trials are pivotal in validating and refining decision-making algorithms in NO-RT. While structured frameworks such as the NOMS system and emerging AI models provide robust theoretical foundations, they require empirical substantiation through clinical data. In this context, well-designed clinical trials offer the concrete evidence needed to translate these theoretical models into practical, patient-centred treatment plans. This integration of trial outcomes into decision-making processes not only enhances clinical confidence but also ensures that treatment recommendations are underpinned by rigorous, real-world evidence (Kisia, 2025).

WHEN SURGERY ALONE IS NOT ENOUGH—THE ROLE OF RADIATION THERAPY IN CLOSE MARGIN CASES

In oncologic surgery, achieving clear resection margins is crucial to minimize the risk of local recurrence. However, when margins are close—typically defined as less than 2 mm—there is an increased risk of residual disease. For instance, in breast-conserving surgery, close or positive margins have been associated with higher rates of local recurrence, underscoring the need for additional therapy such as radiation (Chae & Min, 2022). Guidelines recommend a minimum margin of 2 mm to reduce the risk of ipsilateral breast tumour recurrence (IBTR). Margins smaller than this threshold may necessitate re-excision or adjuvant RT to ensure local control (Morrow et al., 2016).

MULTIDISCIPLINARY DECISION-MAKING—TUMOR BOARD DISCUSSIONS

Multidisciplinary tumour boards (MTBs) are integral to the decision-making process in oncology, especially in complex cases involving close surgical margins. These boards bring together specialists from surgery, radiation oncology, medical oncology, pathology and radiology to collaboratively determine the optimal treatment plan (Okasako & Bernstein, 2022).

For example, in a study involving patients with close margins, MTB discussions led to the consensus that all such patients should receive RT to the primary tumour bed, with doses ranging from 60 to 65 Gy. Chemotherapy was considered only for those with additional high-risk features, such as extracapsular nodal spread (Okasako & Bernstein, 2022).

The collaborative approach of MTBs ensures that treatment decisions are tailored to the individual patient's risk profile, balancing the benefits of additional therapy against potential side effects. This is particularly important in cases where the evidence for adjuvant treatments like RT may be discordant, necessitating nuanced discussions among the care team (Machado et al., 2023). When surgical margins are close, the integration of RT into the treatment plan is often essential to achieve optimal oncologic outcomes. MTBs play a critical role in evaluating these cases, ensuring that decisions are evidence based and personalized to each patient's unique clinical scenario.

DETAILED OVERVIEW OF KEY TRIALS—TARGIT-A TRIAL

One of the most influential studies in the realm of NO-RT is the TARGIT-A trial. This trial was designed to assess the efficacy of intraoperative radiotherapy (IORT) as an alternative to traditional whole-breast radiotherapy in patients with early-stage breast cancer. The study carefully selected patients based on stringent criteria to ensure that only those with early-stage disease were included, allowing for a precise evaluation of IORT's impact on local recurrence rates. The key finding from this trial was that IORT demonstrated non-inferiority compared to standard radiotherapy, thereby validating its potential as a viable NO-RT approach (Kisia, 2025).

IMPACT ON DECISION-MAKING

The practical implications of the TARGIT-A trial are significant. Its findings have been directly integrated into clinical decision-making tools, such as decision trees and risk stratification models. These tools assist clinicians by mapping patient-specific risk profiles against trial outcomes, ultimately guiding the selection of appropriate treatment modalities. By embedding the trial's evidence into these algorithms, practitioners can more accurately determine which patients may safely forego traditional RT without compromising treatment efficacy. This patient-centred approach minimizes unnecessary exposure to radiation and underscores the importance of evidence-based decision-making in NO-RT (Kisia, 2025).

ADDITIONAL TRIALS AND COMPARATIVE ANALYSIS

Beyond the TARGIT-A trial, other significant clinical studies have contributed valuable insights into NO-RT. For instance, the PULS-Pal trial has examined personalized ultra-fractionated stereotactic adaptive RT, focusing on patients with palliative head and neck cancers. This trial primarily evaluated local control and the safety profile of reduced or alternative radiation strategies, offering critical data for tailoring treatment in a palliative context (Courtney et al., 2024).

A comparative analysis of these trials reveals both commonalities and key differences. While TARGIT-A concentrated on early-stage breast cancer and established the non-inferiority of IORT, the PULS-Pal trial addressed the challenges inherent in palliative care, emphasizing individualized treatment protocols. Both trials share a commitment to patient-centred approaches and underscore the importance of precise patient selection. However, their methodologies differ significantly; TARGIT-A's randomized controlled design provided robust evidence for a specific therapeutic alternative, whereas PULS-Pal's adaptive approach highlights the evolving nature of RT in complex clinical scenarios. This diversity in trial design and patient focus enriches the overall decision-making framework in NO-RT, providing clinicians with a more nuanced understanding of when and how to apply non-radiation strategies effectively (Rinderknecht et al., 2024).

Major clinical trials such as TARGIT-A and PULS-Pal play an essential role in refining decision-making algorithms in NO-RT. By providing empirical evidence that complements structured frameworks and AI models, these trials ensure that treatment decisions are both scientifically robust and tailored to individual patient needs. The integration of trial data into decision trees and risk stratification models ultimately enhances clinical practice by promoting personalized, evidence-based care (Courtney et al., 2024; Rinderknecht et al., 2024; Kisia, 2025).

CLINICAL TRIALS SUPPORTING NO-RT

De-escalation trials, including prominent studies like the LUMINA trial, have advanced our understanding of when RT may be safely omitted in certain patient populations. However, these trials often come with significant limitations that restrict the generalizability of their findings. One key limitation is the use of stringent inclusion and exclusion criteria that can inadvertently narrow the study population. For example, the LUMINA trial specifically excluded younger women—typically those under 40 years of age—thereby limiting the applicability of its results to a broader spectrum of breast cancer patients (Whelan et al., 2023). This exclusion raises concerns about whether the favourable outcomes observed in the trial can be extended to younger patients, who may have different tumour biology and treatment responses.

Another limitation is the underrepresentation of diverse demographic groups, including racial and ethnic minorities. Many de-escalation studies are conducted in specific geographic regions or within populations that do not reflect the broader patient community. This lack of diversity means that the trial outcomes might not be applicable to all groups, particularly if genetic, socioeconomic or environmental factors influence treatment efficacy (Smith et al., 2015). Furthermore, patients with significant comorbidities or those who present with more aggressive disease characteristics are often excluded from these trials. As a result, the findings tend to favour a select group of patients with inherently better prognosis, which can skew the perceived benefits of a de-escalated treatment approach.

Additionally, the short-term follow-up in some trials limits our understanding of long-term outcomes and late toxicities. While de-escalation trials may demonstrate immediate benefits in terms of reduced side effects and improved quality of life, the potential for late recurrences or unexpected complications cannot be fully assessed without extended follow-up periods (Mehanna et al., 2020).

Overall, the limitations of de-escalation trials underscore the need for further research that includes a more representative sample of patients. Future studies should strive to incorporate diverse demographic groups and longer follow-up durations to ensure that treatment recommendations are equitable and applicable across all patient populations (Mehanna et al., 2020). Addressing these limitations is essential to advancing personalized cancer care and ensuring that all patients benefit from optimized, evidence-based treatment strategies.

ETHICAL CONSIDERATIONS IN RT DE-ESCALATION

The shift toward NO-RT and de-escalation protocols in cancer treatment raises significant ethical challenges. As healthcare providers strive to balance treatment efficacy with the reduction of unnecessary radiation exposure, complex ethical dilemmas emerge. These dilemmas are compounded by issues related to patient autonomy, informed consent and legal accountability when treatment deviations lead to adverse outcomes.

Ethical Dilemmas in NO-RT

One of the most challenging ethical questions arises when patients, particularly elderly individuals, decline RT despite its potential survival benefits. In cases where the evidence supports a survival advantage with the inclusion of RT, physicians face a dilemma: respecting a patient's autonomy versus their duty to recommend the best available treatment. For instance, an elderly patient with early-stage lung cancer may choose to decline RT due to concerns over quality of life or the perceived burden of treatment. While respecting their decision is ethically imperative, clinicians must also consider the potential consequences of omitting a treatment that could improve survival. This raises a critical ethical issue: Should doctors continue to recommend RT for survival benefits, even if the patient declines, or should they prioritize the patient's right to refuse treatment? The tension between beneficence (the duty to act in the patient's best interest) and respect for autonomy remains at the forefront of such cases.

Informed Consent and Shared Decision-Making

The principle of informed consent is central to the ethical practice of NO-RT. Patients must be fully informed about the potential risks and benefits of both receiving and forgoing RT. Shared decision-making models encourage dialogue between the clinician and patient, ensuring that the patient's values and preferences are integrated into the treatment plan. In practice, this means that when a patient declines RT, the clinician should document the discussion thoroughly, including an explanation of how RT might enhance survival outcomes and reduce recurrence risks. However, even with robust informed consent, ethical quandaries persist, especially when subsequent outcomes such as tumour recurrence or metastasis are observed.

Legal Implications and Malpractice Claims

The ethical considerations of de-escalation are not confined to patient–physician dynamics; they also extend into the legal realm. Legal cases have surfaced where the omission of RT in certain cancer treatments has led to malpractice claims. A notable example comes from the UK, where a case involving cervical cancer highlighted the potential legal risks of de-escalation. In this instance, a patient with cervical cancer was managed under a NO-RT protocol.

Unfortunately, the omission of RT contributed to a recurrence of the disease, ultimately leading to a lawsuit against the treating institution. The plaintiffs argued that the standard of care was not met and that RT should have been administered to prevent disease progression. This case underscores the legal vulnerability associated with NO-RT, particularly when de-escalation protocols are not supported by universally accepted clinical guidelines.

Balancing Risk and Benefit

In de-escalation trials and NO-RT protocols, a thorough risk–benefit analysis is crucial. Clinicians must weigh the potential benefits of reducing radiation exposure such as decreased toxicity, improved quality of life and lower long-term side effects against the risk of inadequate local control and subsequent tumour recurrence. These considerations become even more complicated when demographic factors, such as age and comorbidities, are involved. For example, while older patients may prioritize quality of life over marginal survival benefits, younger patients might accept higher toxicity risks in exchange for improved long-term outcomes. The ethical imperative is to tailor treatment recommendations to the individual patient's clinical context, ensuring that decisions are both evidence based and aligned with patient values.

REAL-WORLD DATA ON NO-RT IMPLEMENTATION

The adoption of NO-RT protocols has been a transformative approach in cancer care, with significant implementations observed in various healthcare settings. Denmark, in particular, has been at the forefront of integrating real-world data (RWD) into clinical practice, leading to substantial reductions in unnecessary radiation exposure and improved patient outcomes.

Reduction in Radiation Exposure

One of the most notable successes of NO-RT protocols in Denmark is the marked reduction in radiation exposure. By leveraging RWD, clinicians have been able to align treatment decisions with the latest evidence-based practices. In Denmark, the implementation of NO-RT strategies has resulted in fewer patients receiving RT when it is not clinically necessary. This reduction in exposure is crucial, as it minimizes the risk of radiation-induced side effects and long-term complications (Olsson et al., 2025). The Danish experience serves as a model for how data-driven protocols can optimize treatment and improve safety without compromising the quality of care.

Enhanced Patient Outcomes

RWD plays a critical role in monitoring and improving patient outcomes post-implementation of NO-RT protocols. By systematically collecting and analysing patient data, healthcare providers have observed notable improvements in quality of life and treatment efficacy. For example, patients who have been spared unnecessary RT have experienced fewer adverse effects, leading to better overall wellbeing and satisfaction with their treatment plans (Zura et al., 2021). This evidence supports the notion that, for selected patient populations, omitting RT can be a safe and effective strategy that enhances both survival and quality of life.

Data-Driven Decision-Making

The integration of RWD into clinical workflows has allowed for a more personalized approach to treatment planning. By combining clinical, genomic and imaging data, AI-driven algorithms can provide a comprehensive view of each patient's unique profile. This holistic perspective enables clinicians to tailor treatment strategies, ensuring that decisions are based on a complete understanding of patient-specific factors (Liu & Panagiotakos, 2022). As a result, treatment plans can be optimized not only for efficacy but also for resource allocation, thereby enhancing the overall efficiency of healthcare delivery.

INTEGRATION INTO DECISION-MAKING MODELS

The use of RWD is essential in developing robust decision-making models and algorithms that inform NO-RT protocols. Machine learning applications have been at the forefront of this integration, with advanced algorithms predicting treatment outcomes such as time to treatment discontinuation. These predictive models enable clinicians to forecast patient responses and adjust treatment plans accordingly (Meng et al., 2022). Furthermore, by analysing RWD at the population level, decision-making models can be refined to reflect specific demographic responses to treatments, ensuring that clinical guidelines are more relevant and tailored to diverse patient groups.

Regulatory bodies have also begun to recognize the value of RWD in shaping evidence-based policies and practices. The increasing regulatory acceptance of RWD underscores its potential to inform clinical decisions and drive policy changes that favour personalized medicine (Zura et al., 2021). This trend is paving the way for broader adoption of NO-RT protocols, where treatment decisions are continuously refined based on emerging data.

Challenges and Future Directions

Despite the clear advantages, several challenges persist in the widespread implementation of RWD-driven NO-RT protocols. Data quality and privacy concerns remain significant obstacles, requiring ongoing refinement of data collection and analysis methodologies (Zura et al., 2021). Additionally, integrating disparate data sources into coherent, actionable insights is an area that demands further research and collaboration among healthcare institutions, technology developers and regulatory agencies.

In conclusion, the real-world implementation of NO-RT protocols, particularly in settings like Denmark, demonstrates the profound impact of integrating RWD into clinical practice. By reducing unnecessary radiation exposure, enhancing patient outcomes and enabling data-driven decision-making, NO-RT protocols represent a significant advancement in personalized cancer care. As challenges related to data quality and integration are addressed, the potential for these protocols to become standard practice across broader patient populations will continue to grow, ultimately leading to more effective and safer treatment strategies for cancer patients.

ALGORITHM DEVELOPMENT

Integration of Clinical Data

Algorithms are increasingly being built upon data derived from clinical trials, incorporating key metrics such as the number needed to treat (NNT) and time-to-benefit (TTB) values. These quantitative indicators are critical for tailoring treatment strategies to individual patients (Alsalemi et al., 2024). By embedding clinical trial data into statistical models, clinicians can better predict patient outcomes and adjust therapies accordingly, making the entire decision-making process more evidence driven.

Machine Learning Applications

The evolution of machine learning has further enriched algorithm development. Regression models and neural networks have been utilized to sift through large datasets and generate predictive analytics that forecast patient responses with high accuracy. These models support clinicians by filtering through complex variables to offer recommendations that are not only data driven but also adapt over time as more patient data become available.

Clinical Decision Trees

Another critical development is the implementation of clinical decision trees (CDTs). CDTs enhance the interpretability and transparency of algorithmic recommendations. By mapping out the decision-making process in a step-by-step manner, these trees make it easier for clinicians to understand and trust the underlying logic of the recommendations (Ebben et al., 2024). The structured nature of decision trees supports a more systematic approach to patient care, ensuring that decision nodes are clearly defined and grounded in trial-derived data.

IMPLICATIONS FOR CLINICAL PRACTICE

Evidence-Based Practice and Reduction of Cognitive Bias

One of the primary advantages of integrating trial-derived data into clinical algorithms is the reinforcement of evidence-based practice. Validated decision-making models help minimize cognitive bias by standardizing treatment recommendations based on empirical evidence rather than subjective judgment (Alsalemi et al., 2024). This standardization is crucial in fostering consistent, high-quality patient care and in supporting clinical decisions that are transparent and replicable.

Enhanced Patient Outcomes

The personalized nature of these algorithms means that individual patient characteristics are thoroughly considered when formulating treatment plans. This tailored approach has been shown to enhance overall patient outcomes, ensuring that each treatment decision is optimized for effectiveness and efficiency (Ojo & Kiobel, 2024).

Limitations and Future Directions

Despite significant advancements, challenges remain. Data bias and privacy concerns continue to limit the widespread adoption of these models (Ojo & Kiobel, 2024). There is also a need for further research to refine predictive models and address ethical considerations, which will ultimately lead to even more robust and inclusive algorithms.

CLINICAL PATHWAYS—DETAILED PATHWAYS INTEGRATING NO RADIATION THERAPY INTO STANDARD TREATMENT PROTOCOLS

Clinical pathways including NO-RT in the standard protocols of oncology are important for optimization of patient care. These pathways are mainly to standardize the treatment method by fostering multidisciplinary collaborations and improving patient outcomes using evidence-based streamlined approaches.

High-risk paediatric oncology patients, especially those with oncologic emergencies like hyperleukocytosis, benefited significantly from clinical pathways. These structural frameworks help in collaboration and timely intervention for the reduction of mortality and morbidity (Reschke et al., 2022). Specific pathways for conditions like hyperleukocytosis and anterior mediastinal masses ensure comprehensive and immediate care. This shows the importance of personalized pathways for addressing patient needs efficiently.

Clinical pathways also play a critical role in the standardization of breast cancer patients. One of the studies in which the implementation of pathways for nodal RT in patients with positive sentinel lymph node biopsies was explored has improved adherence to evidence-based practices (Gebhardt et al., 2018). By reducing unnecessary variations, these pathways ensure uniform treatment delivery that can ultimately improve patient outcomes and streamline care processes.

Management of pain is another critical factor for cancer. This is particularly true in conditions such as non-small cell lung cancer (NSCLC). One of the systemic reviews has observed a gap in high-level evidence supporting non-radiation pain relief strategies. This shows the need for standardized clinical pathways (Brouns et al., 2020). The development of such pathways can help in guiding early interventions. This ensures effective pain relief is integrated into standard protocols and improves the quality of life for patients. For a visual overview, please refer to **Figure 6.1**.

The clinical pathway development is mainly involved in designing structured care models for addressing patient populations. For example, in a study, the pathways that target bone metastasis have improved adherence to single-fraction RT that has compliance rates rising significantly from 18% to 48% after implementation (Rotenstein et al., 2017). Similarly, in breast cancer, care modification in pathways has increased the utilization of hypo-fractionated whole-breast irradiation from 8.3% to over 75%. This demonstrates their impact on treatment adherence (Chapman et al., 2015; Rajagopalan et al., 2015).

Despite the benefits, the integration of clinical pathways into various healthcare settings presents challenges. Local practices, resource availability and patient needs must be carefully considered to ensure these pathways provide improved care delivery (Bosserman et al., 2021). Additionally, while clinical pathways promote standardization, they may inadvertently limit personalized treatment approaches. This highlights the need for a balance between structured protocols and individualized care. Clinical pathways integrating NO-RT into oncology protocols are essential for advancing patient care. These pathways foster evidence-based treatment, enhance multidisciplinary collaboration and improve patient outcomes. However, their successful implementation requires ongoing evaluation

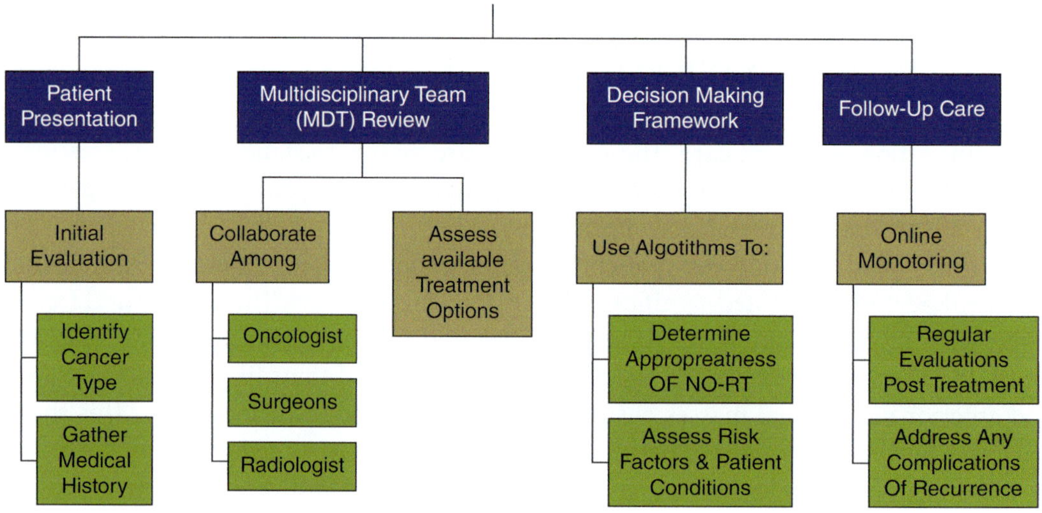

FIGURE 6.1 Clinical pathways integrating NO-RT.

and adaptation to emerging evidence and patient needs, ensuring they complement rather than constrain care delivery. By addressing these challenges, clinical pathways can remain an indispensable tool in modern oncology.

CUSTOMIZATION OF CARE—TAILORING TREATMENT PLANS BASED ON THE INDIVIDUAL PATIENT

The customization of care in cancer treatment mainly without RT shows the significance of developing treatment plans that are tailored to the individual characteristics of patients. This approach combines advanced technologies and methods for improving treatment efficiency and also reduces adverse effects.

AI is transforming cancer care by leveraging multi-omics data and electronic health records (EHRs) for the prediction of optimal treatment paths. This ensures tailored interventions and improvements in patient outcomes. AI frameworks like machine learning models can help in analysing complex datasets for the identification of biomarkers that are critical to therapy response. For example, methods like random forests and convolutional neural networks (CNNs) help in refining treatment decisions for patients with specific cancer subtypes (Vegesna, 2024). These technologies enable clinicians to match patients with the most effective therapies. This helps in promoting precision medicine in terms of NO-RT.

Precision medicine mainly relies on the genetic testing method that helps in the identification of mutations and molecular markers. This guides treatment decisions and improves therapeutic outcomes. The molecular subtyping in breast cancer has led to the development of targeted therapies. Some of the therapies are hormonal treatments for receptor-positive tumours and immunotherapy for specific subtypes (Mahmood et al., 2024; Papalexis et al., 2024). The information from these molecular therapies helps clinicians provide alternative therapies that are less invasive compared to radiation. These tailored treatment strategies reflect the unique biological makeup of each patient.

Patient-derived models provide a robust method for testing and refining personalized treatments. Some techniques, like culturing patient-derived tumour explants, help in facilitating the real-time assessment of drug responses that helps clinicians adapt treatment plans to actual tumour behaviour (Louandre et al., 2016). Similarly, high-throughput methods like whole-genome sequencing help in improving the discovery of biomarkers by enhancing the sensitivity and specificity of personalized therapies (Diamandis et al., 2010). These methods provide a foundation for personalized treatment development that can bypass the need for radiation in some cases.

Molecular profiling and predictive modelling play an important role in the creation of personalized care frameworks. Molecular profiling identifies some specific biomarkers and therapeutic targets, and predictive models like Bayesian nonparametric approaches can cluster patients based on their shared predictive characteristics. This integration helps clinicians in selecting the most suitable treatment methods for individual patients (Matchett et al., 2017; Pedone et al., 2022).

Despite the promise of customized care, there are still some challenges that persist. Issues like data security, ethical concerns, cost and disparities in access to advanced treatments limit the widespread adoption of personalized medicine (Minvielle et al., 2021; Waghmare & Khannam, 2024). Moreover, tumour heterogeneity and the complexity of integrating advanced methodologies into existing healthcare systems present significant barriers. Ongoing research aims to address these challenges by integrating AI and nanotechnology to refine treatment strategies further, ensuring equitable outcomes for all patients (Matchett et al., 2017; Mahmood et al., 2024). The customization of care in alternatives to RT show the potential for tailored treatment plans to improve therapeutic efficacy and patient outcomes. However, it is important to address the ethical, financial and systemic challenges to ensure these advancements are accessible and equitable across diverse patient populations.

MONITORING AND FOLLOW-UP—BEST PRACTICES FOR MONITORING PATIENTS WHO UNDERGO NO RADIATION THERAPY

A balance between effective surveillance and minimizing unnecessary procedures is essential for monitoring the patients who undergo NO-RT. The best practice is using personalized treatment methods that can be used as patient-specific risk factors and the nature of cancer. This helps in ensuring optimal results while reducing the burden on patients.

Follow-Up Guidelines

By adhering to risk-based imaging guidelines, effective surveillance can be achieved. The American Urological Association (AUA) recommends some personalized imaging protocols. For low-risk renal cancer patients, computed tomography (CT) or magnetic resonance imaging (MRI) was advised within 3–12 months after surgery. It will be followed by annual imaging for 3 years (Payton, 2013). In the meanwhile, the moderate- to high-risk patients need imaging every 6 months for 3 years. They can then be changed to annual imaging (Payton, 2013). For patients who prefer active surveillance, initial imaging is necessary to determine a baseline tumour growth rate. Also, follow-up biopsy can be used for refining surveillance plans and also for ensuring proper management (Payton, 2013).

PATIENT-CENTRIC APPROACHES

- **Holistic Care:** Best practices extend beyond medical assessments to encompass psychosocial wellbeing. Addressing life post-cancer treatment holistically can enhance overall patient outcomes and quality of life (von Meyenfeldt et al., 2011).

- **Telehealth Options**: Incorporating telehealth options, such as telephone consultations, offers a practical means to reduce the logistical challenges of in-person visits while maintaining high-quality follow-up care (Brada & James, 1995).

Adherence Challenges

- **Real-World Compliance**: Despite well-defined guidelines, real-world adherence remains a significant challenge. Studies report low-compliance rates with surveillance regimens, necessitating less burdensome strategies to enhance patient engagement and improve outcomes (Rubens et al., 2024).

Standard Follow-Up Protocols

Cancer-Specific Strategies

- **Breast Cancer**: Annual imaging remains the cornerstone of follow-up alongside regular history assessments and physical examinations (Ithimakin et al., 2023).
- **Colorectal Cancer**: Biochemical tests, imaging and physical exams are employed, though the optimal frequency and type of surveillance remain under debate (Jeffery et al., 2016; Lauretta et al., 2023).
- **Head and Neck Cancer**: Multidisciplinary follow-up addresses recurrence detection and the management of late adverse effects, emphasizing comprehensive care (Szturz et al., 2020).

Evidence-Based Recommendations

- **Survival and Quality of Life**: While studies indicate that intensive follow-up does not significantly enhance overall survival, it may facilitate the early detection of recurrences, improving patient quality of life (Jeffery et al., 2016; Szturz et al., 2020).
- **Individualized Surveillance**: Surveillance strategies must be personalized, accounting for cancer type, patient history and psychosocial needs (Szturz et al., 2020; Wöll, 2020). Personalized care ensures that monitoring strategies are both effective and patient-centred.

Monitoring patients who undergo NO-RT requires a strategic, evidence-based approach. Best practices prioritize tailored imaging, active surveillance, holistic care and innovative solutions like telehealth to improve outcomes and patient comfort. While intensive follow-up may not yield survival benefits, its role in enhancing quality of life and detecting recurrences underscores the importance of individualized monitoring strategies.

DOCUMENTATION AND DATA COLLECTION—IMPORTANCE OF ROBUST DOCUMENTATION FOR OUTCOME ANALYSIS

Patient-Centric Approaches

Holistic care can be used for the treatment of patients using NO-RT. The best practices that will extend even after the medical assessments are to encompass psychosocial well-being. Overall outcomes of patients and the quality of life can be improved when the post-treatment of cancer is addressed (von Meyenfeldt et al., 2011). Also, telehealth options like telephone consultations provide a practical way to decrease the challenges of in-person visits so maintaining high-quality follow-up care can be done (Brada & James, 1995).

Real-world compliance is more important in patient-centric approaches. Even if there are well-defined guidelines, real-world adherence remains a challenging process. The low rates of compliance with surveillance regimens make it necessary to create a less burdensome approach to improve the engagement of patients and improvement in outcomes (Rubens et al., 2024).

Some other patient-centric approaches are cancer-specific methods. For example, for breast cancer, the annual imaging is an important cornerstone for follow-up. This must be done along with regular assessments of history and physical examinations (Ithimakin et al., 2023). Similarly, for colorectal cancers, biochemical tests, imaging and physical exams are used, even if the optimal frequencies and surveillance type remain unknown (Jeffery et al., 2016; Lauretta et al., 2023). In terms of head and neck cancer, a multidisciplinary follow-up is necessary for addressing the detection of recurrence and managing later adverse effects. This shows the importance of comprehensive care.

EVIDENCE-BASED RECOMMENDATIONS

Studies have indicated that even if intensive follow-up does not significantly improve overall survival, it may help in the early detection of recurrences and improve patient quality of life (Jeffery et al., 2016; Szturz et al., 2020). Surveillance strategies must be personalized for cancer type, patient history and psychosocial needs (Szturz et al., 2020; Wöll, 2020). Personalized care can help in monitoring strategies that are both effective and patient-centred. Monitoring the patients who undergo NO-RT requires a strategic and evidence-based approach. The good methods will prioritize tailored imaging, active surveillance, holistic care and innovative solutions like telehealth to improve outcomes and patient comfort. Even if the intensive follow-up may not provide more survival benefits, it can help in improving the quality of life and detect the recurrence rates, which are important for personalized monitoring approaches.

DOCUMENTATION AND DATA COLLECTION—IMPORTANCE OF ROBUST DOCUMENTATION FOR OUTCOMES ANALYSIS

For the analysis of clinical outcomes, it is necessary to have robust documentation. This is particularly necessary when handling the therapy algorithms without RT. Data integrity can be maintained by accurate documentation, and this will support effective decision-making and also improve the collection of data.

Importance of Documentation

The importance of documentation practices includes data integrity, scientific progress, quality of care and regulatory compliance. The documentation practices like maintenance of a trial master file (TMF) can help in accurately recording the clinical trial information and helps in retrieving it when needed. This approach is important for retrospective studies and helps researchers verify their findings and evaluate the outcomes accurately (Sun & Wei, 2015). Precise documentation can help in research processes that help maintain scientific integrity. This allows for improvements in further studies. Systematically obtaining every aspect of the clinical protocol and outcomes and documenting it can provide a foundation for evidence-based advancements (Antonakos et al., 2002). Precise documentation can also help in improving communication among healthcare providers. This helps in ensuring that treatment plans can be developed according to patient information. This will lead to improved continuity of care and better patient outcomes (Biswas & Talukdar, 2024).

Proper documentation is essential for meeting healthcare regulations and standards. Regular regulatory compliance helps in the maintenance of institutional credibility and has effects on funding opportunities. This reinforces the importance of robust documentation practices (Biswas & Talukdar, 2024).

Data Collection Mechanisms

Data collection can be carried out using various methods that include EHRs and registries. These methods can help in gathering outcome data systematically. These are considered essential for measuring the effectiveness of the treatment and identifying trends that can help in informing future clinical decisions (Carberry, 2023). Combining the data from patients and providers can help in increasing the evaluation of care quality. This is a dual-purpose approach that helps clinicians to make informed decisions. It provides a comprehensive view of therapy effectiveness and patient satisfaction (Whitaker et al., 2018).

Data Integration and Analysis

Combining the data from various sources can help in the analysis of risk factors that are influencing cancer outcomes. However, these factors are commonly documented poorly in current research. This shows the need for improved data collection practices (Zhang et al., 2019; Zhang et al., 2020). Using structured documentation workflows can help streamline data collection. This reduces manual errors and improves the efficiency of clinical trials. Automated systems also support improvements in quality initiatives and increase the timelines of research (Yalamanchi et al., 2022).

CHALLENGES AND CONSIDERATIONS

Despite the benefits, some challenges still persist that limit the achievement of interoperability and standardization across different healthcare systems. This may be due to cost considerations, and it may affect the efficacy of documentation efforts (Tsai et al., 2019). Also, making sure of the completeness of data and accuracy in NO-RT effects needs efforts for training staff and implementing standard protocols. Robust documentation is critical for effective analysis of outcomes mainly in the context of therapy algorithms without any RT. This helps in ensuring the integrity of data that in turn improve the quality of care and also support regulatory compliance. The proper and accurate documentation helps in laying the groundwork to improve patient outcomes. The integration of various data sources and adherence to standardized protocols are necessary to advance clinical practices and improve scientific progress.

EXAMPLES OF HOW ALGORITHMS STREAMLINE NO-RT DECISION-MAKING

The advancement of AI and machine learning in oncology has led to the development of decision-making algorithms that optimize patient management by identifying individuals who can safely avoid RT. These algorithms improve clinical efficiency, minimize unnecessary interventions and enhance patient outcomes by tailoring treatment strategies to individual risk profiles. The following examples illustrate how algorithms are streamlining NO-RT decision-making across various cancer types (Sun et al., 2022).

Breast Cancer Decision-Making Algorithm

For early-stage breast cancer patients, a sophisticated algorithm integrates nanogram assessments to identify individuals who do not require postmastectomy radiation therapy (PMRT). This algorithm, developed by Tang et al. (2020), relies on molecular and pathological data to assess recurrence risks and determine whether RT can be safely omitted. By leveraging predictive analytics, oncologists can focus their attention on high-risk patients while allowing low-risk individuals to avoid the side effects and costs associated with RT. This approach has led to more personalized treatment plans, reduced overtreatment and improved quality of life for patients.

Head and Neck Cancer Risk Assessment Algorithm

The ω score nomogram algorithm for head and neck cancer has proven to be a valuable tool in determining the necessity of RT. Developed by Vitzthum et al. (2020), this algorithm calculates patient-specific risk scores using clinical, histological and genetic markers. Patients with a low recurrence risk may not derive significant benefits from aggressive treatments like RT. Instead, these individuals can be managed with alternative, less invasive therapies, thereby reducing treatment-associated morbidity. This algorithm supports precision medicine by enabling oncologists to tailor treatment intensity based on individualized risk profiles, ensuring optimal patient care while preventing unnecessary radiation exposure.

Rectal Cancer Pathway Algorithm

A clinical pathway algorithm for rectal cancer is transforming treatment decisions by identifying patients who achieve a complete response to neoadjuvant therapy and can safely forego surgery and RT. According to Marincaş et al. (2015), this algorithm evaluates tumour regression grade, imaging results and clinical response markers to assess which patients can be managed through a "watch-and-wait" approach instead of aggressive surgical and radiation interventions. This decision-making tool optimizes resource allocation, reduces complications and enhances patient quality of life by minimizing the burden of treatment while maintaining oncological safety.

Cytoreductive Surgery Decision Algorithm

In cases where patients undergo cytoreductive surgery, an algorithm has been developed to assess tumour characteristics and predict the need for RT. Sammartino et al. (2015) introduced a structured decision model that evaluates factors such as tumour histology, surgical margins and molecular profiles to determine whether RT is necessary postoperatively. By using this evidence-based approach, clinicians can avoid unnecessary radiation exposure in patients with favourable tumour biology, reducing potential toxicity while ensuring optimal treatment outcomes. This algorithm has streamlined patient selection processes, contributing to improved survival rates and reduced treatment-related side effects.

The Role of AI and Machine Learning in NO-RT Decision-Making

Beyond individual algorithms, the integration of AI and machine learning models in oncology is revolutionizing NO-RT decision-making. These models continuously learn from vast datasets, refining their predictive accuracy over time. AI-driven algorithms incorporate real-world evidence, genomic data and treatment outcomes to enhance decision-making precision. As a result, oncologists are increasingly equipped with powerful tools that aid in selecting patients who can safely avoid RT while maintaining oncologic control (Manjunath et al., 2019).

CONCLUSION

The structured decision-making frameworks integrate evidence-based algorithms, especially in terms of NO-RT. AI-driven systems and clinical information are used to optimize patient outcomes and also minimize treatment-related risks. By using tools like the NOMS framework and advanced AI systems like ARCliDS, clinicians can systematically evaluate patient-specific factors and tailor treatment plans to individual needs. The combination of clinical algorithms improves objectivity and also reduces biases in decision-making. This enables more precise identification of candidates for NO-RT. The role of personalized medicine is to utilize genomic and molecular profiling to guide therapy. Additionally, it highlights the transformative potential of AI and machine learning in refining recommendations and improving treatment efficacy. While these frameworks and tools represent significant advancements, the complexity of oncology necessitates a balance between algorithmic precision and clinical judgment. The chapter concludes by emphasizing the importance of adopting evidence-based, patient-centred approaches to maximize the benefits of NO-RT. This structured approach ensures improved patient care, reducing unnecessary interventions and aligning with evolving clinical evidence and technologies.

REFERENCES

Alsalemi, N., Sadowski, C., Elftouh, N., Kilpatrick, K., Houle, S., Leclerc, S., Fernandez, N., & Lafrance, J.-P. (2024). Designing and validating a clinical decision support algorithm for diabetic nephroprotection in older patients. *BMJ Health & Care Informatics*, *31*(1), e100869. https://doi.org/10.1136/bmjhci-2023-100869

Antonakos, C. L., Miller, J. M., & Caruso, C. C. (2002). Critical elements of documentation for data-based research. *Western Journal of Nursing Research*, *24*(1), 87–100. https://doi.org/10.1177/01939450222045725

Bilsky, M. H., & Azeem, S. (2007). The NOMS framework for decision making in metastatic cervical spine tumors. *Current Opinion in Orthopaedics*, *18*(3), 263–269. https://doi.org/10.1097/BCO.0b013e3280d942fc

Biswas, A., & Talukdar, W. (2024). Enhancing clinical documentation with synthetic data: Leveraging generative models for improved accuracy. *International Journal of Innovative Science and Research Technology (IJISRT)*, 1553–1566. https://doi.org/10.38124/ijisrt/IJISRT24MAY2085

Bosserman, L. D., Cianfrocca, M., Yuh, B., Yeon, C., Chen, H., Sentovich, S., Polverini, A., Zachariah, F., Deaville, D., Lee, A. B., Sedrak, M. S., King, E., Gray, S., Morse, D., Glaser, S., Bhatt, G., Adeimy, C., Tan, T., Chao, J., … Johnson, D. (2021). Integrating academic and community cancer care and research through multidisciplinary oncology pathways for value-based care: A review and the city of hope experience. *Journal of Clinical Medicine*, *10*(2), 188. https://doi.org/10.3390/jcm10020188

Brada, M., & James, N. D. (1995). Phone clinic provides excellent support. *BMJ*, *310*(6981), 738–738. https://doi.org/10.1136/bmj.310.6981.738

Brouns, A. J. W. M., De Bie, B. H., Van Den Beuken-van Everdingen, M. H. J., Dingemans, A.-M. C., & Hendriks, L. E. L. (2020). Non-radiation based early pain relief treatment options for patients with non-small cell lung cancer and cancer induced bone pain: A systematic review. *Frontiers in Oncology*, *10*, 509297. https://doi.org/10.3389/fonc.2020.509297

Carberry, K. E. (2023). *How to Measure Health Outcomes: A Hands-on Guide to Getting Started* (1st ed.). Cambridge University Press. https://doi.org/10.1017/9781009240925

Chae, S., & Min, S. Y. (2022). Association of surgical margin status with oncologic outcome in patients treated with breast-conserving surgery. *Current Oncology (Toronto, Ont.)*, *29*(12), 9271–9283. https://doi.org/10.3390/curroncol29120726

Chapman, B. V., Rajagopalan, M. S., Heron, D. E., Flickinger, J. C., & Beriwal, S. (2015). Clinical pathways: A catalyst for the adoption of hypofractionation for early-stage breast cancer. *International Journal of Radiation Oncology*Biology*Physics*, *93*(4), 854–861. https://doi.org/10.1016/j.ijrobp.2015.08.013

Courtney, P. T., L. Santoso, M., Savjani, R. R., K. Reddy, V., Chai-Ho, W., Velez Velez, M. A., J. Wong, D., Palodichuk, C., Basehart, T. V., P. O'Connell, D., Cao, M., Telesca, D., & Chin, R. K. (2024). A phase II study of personalized ultrafractionated stereotactic adaptive radiotherapy for palliative head and neck cancer treatment (PULS-Pal): A single-arm clinical trial protocol. *BMC Cancer*, *24*(1), 1564. https://doi.org/10.1186/s12885-024-13303-5

Dennstädt, F., Treffers, T., Iseli, T., Panje, C., & Putora, P. M. (2021). Creation of clinical algorithms for decision-making in oncology: An example with dose prescription in radiation oncology. *BMC Medical Informatics and Decision Making*, *21*(1), 212. https://doi.org/10.1186/s12911-021-01568-w

Diamandis, M., White, N. M. A., & Yousef, G. M. (2010). Personalized medicine: Marking a new epoch in cancer patient management. *Molecular Cancer Research*, *8*(9), 1175–1187. https://doi.org/10.1158/1541-7786.MCR-10-0264

Ebben, K. C. W. J., Van Vegchel, T., Massa, M., Sloep, M., & Van Der Werf, J. (2024). Development and implementation of clinical decision algorithms for oncology. In J. Mantas, A. Hasman, G. Demiris, K. Saranto, M. Marschollek, T. N. Arvanitis, I. Ognjanović, A. Benis, P. Gallos, E. Zoulias & E. Andrikopoulou (Eds.), *Studies in Health Technology and Informatics*. IOS Press. https://doi.org/10.3233/SHTI240662

Esserman, L. J., Alvarado, M. D., Howe, R. J., Mohan, A. J., Harrison, B., Park, C., O'Donoghue, C., & Ozanne, E. M. (2014). Application of A decision analytic framework for adoption of clinical trial results: Are the data regarding TARGIT-A IORT ready for prime time? *Breast Cancer Research and Treatment*, *144*(2), 371–378. https://doi.org/10.1007/s10549-014-2881-2

Gebhardt, B. J., Thomas, J., Horne, Z. D., Champ, C. E., Ahrendt, G. M., Diego, E., Heron, D. E., & Beriwal, S. (2018). Standardization of nodal radiation therapy through changes to a breast cancer clinical pathway throughout a large, integrated cancer center network. *Practical Radiation Oncology*, *8*(1), 4–12. https://doi.org/10.1016/j.prro.2017.07.012

Ithimakin, S., Luengwatthanakit, N., & Wongkraisri, C. (2023). Follow-up strategies and detection of recurrent breast cancer in the modern era. *Asian Pacific Journal of Cancer Prevention, 24*(4), 1359–1366. https://doi.org/10.31557/APJCP.2023.24.4.1359

Jeffery, M., Hickey, B. E., Hider, P. N., & See, A. M. (2016). Follow-up strategies for patients treated for non-metastatic colorectal cancer. *Cochrane Database of Systematic Reviews*. https://doi.org/10.1002/14651858.CD002200.pub3

Kisia, N. (2025). Abstract A007: Artificial intelligence in radiation therapy: Bringing in a new era of cancer therapy, accurate and fast. *Clinical Cancer Research, 31*(2_Supplement), A007. https://doi.org/10.1158/1557-3265.TARGETEDTHERAP-A007

Lauretta, A., Montori, G., & Guerrini, G. P. (2023). Surveillance strategies following curative resection and non-operative approach of rectal cancer: How and how long? Review of current recommendations. *World Journal of Gastrointestinal Surgery, 15*(2), 177–192. https://doi.org/10.4240/wjgs.v15.i2.177

Lin, F. P. Y. (2020). Design and implementation of an intelligent framework for supporting evidence-based treatment recommendations in precision oncology. https://doi.org/10.1101/2020.11.15.383448

Liu, F., & Panagiotakos, D. (2022). Real-world data: A brief review of the methods, applications, challenges and opportunities. *BMC Medical Research Methodology, 22*(1), 287. https://doi.org/10.1186/s12874-022-01768-6

Louandre, C., Donnadieu, J., Lachaier, E., Page, C., Chauffert, B., & Galmiche, A. (2016). Personalization of the medical treatment of solid tumours using patient-derived tumour explants (Review). *International Journal of Oncology, 48*(3), 895–899. https://doi.org/10.3892/ijo.2016.3345

Machado, L. B., Brody, M. B., Rotenberg, S. E., Stachelek, G. C., & Fernandez, J. G. (2023). Breast cancer tumor board: A radiologist's guide to postmastectomy radiation therapy. *RadioGraphics, 43*(3), e220086. https://doi.org/10.1148/rg.220086

Mahmood, A. R., Jha, D. A. M., & Manivannan, K. (2024). Precision medicine: Personalizing the fight against cancer. *International Journal of Trends in OncoScience, 2*(1), 10–18. https://doi.org/10.22376/ijtos.2023.2.1.10-18

Manjunath, R. B., Shashanka, B. S., Thanukumar, T. N., Arunkumar, B, C., & Nandini, P. (2019). Medical documentation of clinical data and disease prediction. *International Journal of Advance Research and Innovative Ideas in Education, 5*(2), 2865–2871.

Marincaş, A. M., Prunoiu, V. M., Brătucu, E., Cirimbei, C., Ionescu, S., Buzatu, R., & Straja, N. D. (2015). Clinical and paraclinical criteria of patient selection for the non- operative treatment in completely responsive rectal cancer (after neoadjuvant radiochemotherapy). *Chirurgia (Bucharest, Romania: 1990), 110*(4), 351–355.

Matchett, K., Lynam-Lennon, N., Watson, R., & Brown, J. (2017). Advances in precision medicine: Tailoring individualized therapies. *Cancers, 9*(11), 146. https://doi.org/10.3390/cancers9110146

Mehanna, H., Rischin, D., Wong, S. J., Gregoire, V., Ferris, R., Waldron, J., Le, Q.-T., Forster, M., Gillison, M., Laskar, S., Tahara, M., Psyrri, A., Vermorken, J., & Porceddu, S. (2020). De-escalation after de-escalate and RTOG 1016: A head and neck cancer intergroup framework for future de-escalation studies. *Journal of Clinical Oncology, 38*(22), 2552–2557. https://doi.org/10.1200/JCO.20.00056

Meng, W., Zhang, X., Ru, B., & Guan, Y. (2022). A machine learning approach to real-world time to treatment discontinuation prediction. *Advanced Intelligent Systems, 5*(4). https://doi.org/10.22541/au.166065465.59798123/v1

Minvielle, E., Fourcade, A., Ricketts, T., & Waelli, M. (2021). Current developments in delivering customized care: A scoping review. *BMC Health Services Research, 21*(1), 575. https://doi.org/10.1186/s12913-021-06576-0

Morrow, M., Van Zee, K. J., Solin, L. J., Houssami, N., Chavez-MacGregor, M., Harris, J. R., Horton, J., Hwang, S., Johnson, P. L., Marinovich, M. L., Schnitt, S. J., Wapnir, I., & Moran, M. S. (2016). Society of Surgical Oncology–American Society for Radiation Oncology–American Society of Clinical Oncology consensus guideline on margins for breast-conserving surgery with whole-breast irradiation in ductal carcinoma in situ. *Journal of Clinical Oncology, 34*(33), 4040–4046. https://doi.org/10.1200/JCO.2016.68.3573

Niraula, D., Sun, W., Jin, J., Dinov, I. D., Cuneo, K., Jamaluddin, J., Matuszak, M. M., Luo, Y., Lawrence, T. S., Jolly, S., Ten Haken, R. K., & El Naqa, I. (2023). A clinical decision support system for AI-assisted decision-making in response-adaptive radiotherapy (ARCLiDS). *Scientific Reports, 13*(1), 5279. https://doi.org/10.1038/s41598-023-32032-6

Okasako, J., & Bernstein, C. (2022). Multidisciplinary tumor boards and guiding patient care: The ap role. *Journal of the Advanced Practitioner in Oncology, 13*(3), 227–230. https://doi.org/10.6004/jadpro.2022.13.3.9

Ojo, O. O., & Kiobel, B. (2024). Integrating predictive analytics in clinical trials: A paradigm shift in personalized medicine. *World Journal of Biology Pharmacy and Health Sciences, 19*(3), 308–320. https://doi.org/10.30574/wjbphs.2024.19.3.0630

Olsson, C. E., Krogh, S. L., Karlsson, M., Eriksen, J. G., Björk-Eriksson, T., Grau, C., Norman, D., Offersen, B. V., Nyholm, T., Overgaard, J., Zackrisson, B., & Hansen, C. R. (2025). Danish and Swedish National Data Collections for Cancer—Solutions for radiotherapy. *Clinical Oncology, 37*(1), 103657. https://doi.org/10.1016/j.clon.2024.10.009

Papalexis, P., Georgakopoulou, V., Drossos, P., Thymara, E., Nonni, A., Lazaris, A., Zografos, G., Spandidos, D., Kavantzas, N., & Thomopoulou, G. E. (2024). Precision medicine in breast cancer (Review). *Molecular and Clinical Oncology, 21*(5), 78. https://doi.org/10.3892/mco.2024.2776

Payton, S (2013). New AUA guideline tackles follow-up monitoring of small renal masses. *Nature Reviews Urology, 10*(7), 367–367. https://doi.org/10.1038/nrurol.2013.119

Pedone, M., Argiento, R., & Stingo, F. C. (2022). Personalized treatment selection via product partition models with covariates. *arXiv*. https://doi.org/10.48550/ARXIV.2210.06030

Rajagopalan, M. S., Flickinger, J. C., Heron, D. E., & Beriwal, S. (2015). Changing practice patterns for breast cancer radiation therapy with clinical pathways: An analysis of hypofractionation in a large, integrated cancer center network. *Practical Radiation Oncology, 5*(2), 63–69. https://doi.org/10.1016/j.prro.2014.10.004

Reschke, A., Richards, R. M., Smith, S. M., Long, A. H., Marks, L. J., Schultz, L., Kamens, J. L., Aftandilian, C., Davis, K. L., Gruber, T., & Sakamoto, K. M. (2022). Development of clinical pathways to improve multidisciplinary care of high-risk pediatric oncology patients. *Frontiers in Oncology, 12*, 1033993. https://doi.org/10.3389/fonc.2022.1033993

Ribi, K., Panje, C. M., Thalmann, G. N., Zwahlen, D. R., Früh, M., Thürlimann, B., … Zaman, K. (2022). Towards a novel approach guiding the decision-making for systemic anticancer treatment in far advanced cancer patients: The SACT-PI Decision Framework. *ESMO Open, 7*(3), 100497. https://doi.org/10.1016/j.esmoop.2022.100497

Rinderknecht, E., von Winning, D., Kravchuk, A., Schäfer, C., Schnabel, M. J., Siepmann, S., Mayr, R., Grassinger, J., Goßler, C., Pohl, F., Siska, P. J., Zeman, F., Breyer, J., Schmelzer, A., Gilfrich, C., Brookman-May, S. D., Burger, M., Haas, M., & May, M. (2024). Modification and validation of the System Causability Scale using AI-based therapeutic recommendations for urological cancer patients: A basis for the development of a prospective comparative study. *Current Oncology, 31*(11), 7061–7073. https://doi.org/10.3390/curroncol31110520

Rotenstein, L. S., Hartsell, W. F., & Movsas, B. (2017). Impact of a clinical pathway tool on appropriate palliative radiation therapy for bone metastases. *Practical Radiation Oncology, 7*(1), e1–e7. https://doi.org/10.1016/j.prro.2016.06.003

Rubens, M., Oduyale, O., Eltahir, A., Kim, H., Ohman, K., Wise, P., Hunt, S., Silviera, M., Mutch, M., Glasgow, S. C., Smith, R., & Chapman, W. (2024). "Watch-and-wait" or "lost to follow-up"? Real-world adherence with surveillance for nonoperative management of rectal cancer. https://doi.org/10.21203/rs.3.rs-3940931/v1

Sammartino, P., Accarpio, F., Sollazzo, B. M., Impagnatiello, A., Cornali, T., & Biacchi, D. (2015). Patient selection for treatment. In A. Di Giorgio & E. Pinto (Eds.), *Treatment of Peritoneal Surface Malignancies* (pp. 195–205). Springer Milan. https://doi.org/10.1007/978-88-470-5711-1_13

Smith, J. J., Chow, O. S., Gollub, M. J., Nash, G. M., Temple, L. K., Weiser, M. R., Guillem, J. G., Paty, P. B., Avila, K., & Garcia-Aguilar, J. (2015). Organ preservation in rectal adenocarcinoma: A phase II randomized controlled trial evaluating 3-year disease-free survival in patients with locally advanced rectal cancer treated with chemoradiation plus induction or consolidation chemotherapy, and total mesorectal excision or nonoperative management. *BMC Cancer, 15*(1), 767. https://doi.org/10.1186/s12885-015-1632-z

Sun, H., & Wei, Z. (2015). Documentation archiving in clinical data management. *Yao Xue Xue Bao = Acta Pharmaceutica Sinica, 50*(11), 1410–1414.

Sun, X. (2022). Real-world data and real-world evidence. In W. Zhang, F. Yan, F. Chen, & S. -C. Chow (Eds.), *Advanced Statistics in Regulatory Critical Clinical Initiatives* (1st ed., pp. 105–132). Chapman and Hall/CRC. https://doi.org/10.1201/9781003107323-5

Szturz, P., Van Laer, C., Simon, C., Van Gestel, D., Bourhis, J., & Vermorken, J. B. (2020). Follow-up of head and neck cancer survivors: Tipping the balance of intensity. *Frontiers in Oncology, 10*, 688. https://doi.org/10.3389/fonc.2020.00688

Tang, Y., Zhang, Y.-J., Zhang, N., Shi, M., Wen, G., Cheng, J., Wang, H.-M., Liu, M., Wang, X.-H., Guo, Q.-S., Wu, H.-F., Ma, C.-Y., Jin, J., Liu, Y.-P., Song, Y.-W., Fang, H., Ren, H., Wang, S.-L., & Li, Y.-X. (2020). Nomogram predicting survival as a selection criterion for postmastectomy radiotherapy in patients with T1 to T2 breast cancer with 1 to 3 positive lymph nodes. *Cancer, 126*(S16), 3857–3866. https://doi.org/10.1002/cncr.32963

Tsai, C. J., Riaz, N., & Gomez, S. L. (2019). Big data in cancer research: Real-world resources for precision oncology to improve cancer care delivery. *Seminars in Radiation Oncology, 29*(4), 306–310. https://doi.org/10.1016/j.semradonc.2019.05.002

Vegesna, V. (2024). Ai-driven personalized medicine: A frame work for tailored cancer treatment. *International Journal of Innovative Research in Advanced Engineering, 11*(06), 747–752. https://doi.org/10.26562/ijirae.2024.v1106.06

Vitzthum, L. K., Park, H., Zakeri, K., Bryant, A. K., Feng, C., Shen, H., Cohen, E. E. W., Murphy, J. D., & Mell, L. K. (2020). Selection of head and neck cancer patients for intensive therapy. *International Journal of Radiation Oncology*Biology*Physics, 106*(1), 157–166. https://doi.org/10.1016/j.ijrobp.2019.09.011

von Meyenfeldt, M., Boersma, L., Maessen, J., & Keymeulen, K. (2011). Follow-up in oncology: Focused on the patient and the disease. *Nederlands Tijdschrift Voor Geneeskunde, 155*(45), A4127.

Waghmare, S. G., & Khannam, A. N. Z. (2024). Individualized medicine: Revolutionizing healthcare with tailored therapies. *EPRA International Journal of Research & Development (IJRD)*, 18–20. https://doi.org/10.36713/epra17655

Whelan, T. J., Smith, S., Parpia, S., Fyles, A. W., Bane, A., Liu, F.-F., Rakovitch, E., Chang, L., Stevens, C., Bowen, J., Provencher, S., Théberge, V., Mulligan, A. M., Kos, Z., Akra, M. A., Voduc, K. D., Hijal, T., Dayes, I. S., Pond, G., … Levine, M. N. (2023). Omitting radiotherapy after breast-conserving surgery in luminal a breast cancer. *New England Journal of Medicine, 389*(7), 612–619. https://doi.org/10.1056/NEJMoa2302344

Whitaker, T. J., Mayo, C. S., Ma, D. J., Haddock, M. G., Miller, R. C., Corbin, K. S., Neben-Wittich, M., Leenstra, J. L., Laack, N. N., Fatyga, M., Schild, S. E., Vargas, C. E., Tzou, K. S., Hadley, A. R., Buskirk, S. J., & Foote, R. L. (2018). Data collection of patient outcomes: One institution's experience. *Journal of Radiation Research, 59*(suppl_1), i19–i24. https://doi.org/10.1093/jrr/rry013

Wöll, E. (2020). Evidence-based follow-up. *Memo—Magazine of European Medical Oncology, 13*(1), 5–6. https://doi.org/10.1007/s12254-019-00568-x

Yalamanchi, P., Casper, K. A., Evans, J., Mierzwa, M., Morrison, R. J., Prince, M. E., & Mayo, C. S. (2022). Facilitating automated data analytics through structured head and neck oncology tumor board documentation. *JCO Clinical Cancer Informatics, 6*, e2100168. https://doi.org/10.1200/CCI.21.00168

Zhang, H., Guo, Y., & Bian, J. (2019). Ontology for documentation of variable and data source selection process to support integrative data analysis in cancer outcomes research. SEPDA@ISWC.

Zhang, H., Guo, Y., Prosperi, M., & Bian, J. (2020). An ontology-based documentation of data discovery and integration process in cancer outcomes research. *BMC Medical Informatics and Decision Making, 20*(S4), 292. https://doi.org/10.1186/s12911-020-01270-3

Zura, R., Irwin, D. E., Mack, C. D., Aldridge, M. L., & Mackowiak, J. I. (2021). Real- world evidence: A primer. *Journal of Orthopaedic Trauma, 35*(1), S1–S5. https://doi.org/10.1097/BOT.0000000000002037

CHAPTER 7

Case Studies

Showing Effective Uses of NO-RT Principles

Shrikant Khare, Peeyush Shukla and Shantanu Pawar

CASE STUDY 1

The clinical approach to managing primary mediastinal B-cell lymphoma (PMBCL) has undergone a paradigm shift, with increased emphasis on individualized patient care strategies. This case study is a patient in whom the omission of radiotherapy (no radiotherapy [NO-RT]) was successfully implemented and that led to an excellent clinical outcome.

Patient Demographics and Clinical Presentation

The patient was a 28-year-old female presenting with a 3-month history of progressive dyspnoea, chest pain and fatigue. She did not have any significant past medical history and reported no prior malignancies or cardiac disease. Physical examination showed an anterior mediastinal mass, and this was confirmed by imaging to be 9 cm in diameter. Histological analysis from a mediastinal biopsy showed CD20+, CD30+ and BCL6+ diffuse large B-cell lymphoma consistent with PMBCL.

Initial Treatment Approach

The patient had undergone frontline immunochemotherapy using a DA-EPOCH-R regimen that is a dose-adjusted regimen of etoposide, prednisone, vincristine, cyclophosphamide, doxorubicin and rituximab. This regimen was chosen mainly based on emerging evidence supporting its efficacy in PMBCL and its ability to achieve durable responses. Chemotherapy was administered over six cycles with strict adherence to dose adjustment protocols to reduce the toxicity.

Response Evaluation

Post-treatment response evaluation was performed 5 weeks after the completion of chemotherapy. PET/CT imaging revealed a Deauville Score (DS) of 2. This shows a complete metabolic response (CMR) as per the Lugano classification. No residual hypermetabolic

DOI: 10.1201/9781003529071-7

activity was observed in the mediastinal region. Central review of the PET/CT scans by a panel of nuclear medicine specialists has confirmed these findings.

Decision to Omit Radiotherapy

The decision to omit radiotherapy was based on the IELSG37 trial results. This trial has shown noninferiority in progression-free survival (PFS) and overall survival (OS) for patients achieving CMR who were managed with observation alone. This decision was further supported by the patient's excellent response to chemotherapy and the potential long-term risks associated with mediastinal radiotherapy such as cardiopulmonary toxicity and secondary malignancies.

Follow-Up and Monitoring

The patient was then brought into a structured follow-up protocol. Surveillance included clinical evaluations every 3 months during the first 2 years, semi-annual assessments in years 3–5 and annual visits thereafter. Imaging studies were conducted at 6 months, 1 year and then annually consistent with international guidelines for PMBCL.

Outcome

At the 30-month follow-up, the patient remained in complete remission with no evidence of disease recurrence on PET/CT imaging. The 5-year OS and PFS for patients with similar profiles managed without radiotherapy in the IELSG37 trial were 99% and 96.2%, respectively. This further corroborated the decision to adopt a NO-RT strategy.

Discussion

This case shows the feasibility and success of omitting radiotherapy in select patients with PMBCL who achieve CMR after immunochemotherapy. The IELSG37 trial provided evidence that supports radiotherapy omission in these patients, thus challenging the traditional paradigm of routine consolidation radiotherapy.

The decision-making process in this case shows the importance of combining trial data with patient-specific factors. For this patient, omitting radiotherapy reduced the risk of long-term complications while maintaining excellent disease control. Also, the low absolute risk difference in 30-month PFS between the observation and radiotherapy arms of 0.68% supports the clinical availability in this approach.

Future Directions

This case contributes to the growing body of evidence advocating for a personalized approach to the management of PMBCL. While the omission of radiotherapy is supported for patients achieving CMR, future research should explore biomarkers and imaging modalities that can refine risk stratification and further individualize therapy. Additionally, prospective studies are warranted to evaluate the long-term impact of NO-RT on survival, quality of life and late treatment-related toxicities.

Conclusion

The successful implementation of NO-RT in this case demonstrates the efficacy and safety of observation in patients with PMBCL who achieve CMR after induction immunochemotherapy. This approach not only aligns with evidence-based practice but also addresses the broader goals of reducing treatment-related morbidity and improving patient quality of life. As clinical paradigms continue to evolve, this case reinforces the importance of precision medicine in delivering optimal cancer care.

CASE STUDY 2

The watch-and-wait (W&W) strategy for rectal cancer has been considered a non-invasive alternative for patients who achieve a clinical complete response (cCR) after neoadjuvant chemoradiotherapy (CRT). However, implementing this strategy was difficult. This case study presents a scenario where the W&W strategy was considered but ultimately not employed. This emphasizes the complex interplay of clinical, psychological and logistical factors.

Background

A 56-year-old male patient was diagnosed with stage III rectal adenocarcinoma located within 4 cm of the anal verge. His baseline evaluation included a digital rectal examination, colonoscopy and pelvic magnetic resonance imaging (MRI). This confirmed the tumour's advanced T3N1 stage. After neoadjuvant CRT with capecitabine and a total radiation dose of 50.4 Gy, a re-evaluation showed no palpable tumour on examination, and endoscopic results were consistent with a flat white scar that was suggestive of a cCR. MRI scans showed no residual tumour or suspicious lymph nodes. Based on these findings, the treating team discussed the possibility of adopting the W&W approach.

Clinical Context

The patient was a candidate for the W&W strategy because of the absence of residual disease on all reassessment modalities. Also, the proximity of the tumour to the anal verge presented a significant risk of requiring a permanent colostomy if total mesorectal excision (TME) surgery was carried out. The potential to preserve sphincter function and avoid life-altering surgical outcomes made W&W an attractive option. However, the team faced the difficulty of balancing the benefits of this conservative strategy against the risks of local regrowth and the psychological burden it may cause on the patient. The decision-making process became more difficult as further factors emerged.

Factors Influencing the Decision—Patient-Specific Concerns

The patient had a history of diabetes mellitus and hypertension. These were well controlled but raised concerns about his ability to undergo salvage surgery in the event of local regrowth. Salvage procedures are often more complex than primary surgery and need meticulous planning and carry additional risks. The patient had expressed significant anxiety about the rigorous follow-up protocol needed for the W&W approach. This includes frequent digital rectal examinations, colonoscopies and imaging. He feared the psychological toll of living with uncertainty and the possibility of disease recurrence.

Tumor Characteristics

While the tumour's location increased the likelihood of sphincter preservation with W&W, it also posed challenges. Tumours located near the anal verge have a higher risk of local regrowth, which, although salvageable in most cases, adds complexity to patient management. Although imaging suggested a cCR, subtle irregularities on MRI raised concerns about potential microscopic disease. These findings, while not definitive, introduced doubt regarding the accuracy of the cCR assessment.

Institutional Protocols and Experience

The multidisciplinary team at the treating centre had limited experience with the W&W strategy. While the protocol had been implemented successfully in select cases, the familiarity of the team with managing salvage scenarios was not extensive. The lack of robust institutional data on outcomes for W&W patients further influenced the decision-making process.

Family Preferences and Support

The patient's family strongly advocated for surgery, citing their perception of it as a definitive cure. Their concern about the uncertainty associated with W&W created additional pressure on the patient and the medical team.

Decision and Outcome

After thorough discussions, the team recommended proceeding with TME surgery rather than adopting the W&W strategy. The decision was based on the following considerations: higher perceived risk of local regrowth in the form of a subtle radiological irregularity, along with the tumour's proximity to the anal verge, which increased the likelihood of regrowth that could complicate subsequent management. The patient and his family prioritized peace of mind over sphincter preservation, favouring the certainty of complete surgical removal. Institutional expertise was that given the limited experience with W&W at the centre, the team felt more confident in ensuring optimal outcomes through surgery.

The patient underwent TME with a permanent colostomy. Pathological examination of the surgical specimen revealed no residual tumour and pathological complete response. Postoperatively the patient experienced minor wound complications and that was resolved within 4 weeks.

Conclusion

The W&W strategy represents a paradigm shift in rectal cancer management that provides a less invasive option for carefully selected patients. However, it is not applicable universally. This case shows the complex interplay of clinical, psychological and institutional factors in determining the best course of action. For this patient, the decision to proceed with surgery ensured peace of mind and oncological safety, demonstrating that the most appropriate treatment is one that aligns with both medical evidence and individual patient circumstances.

LESSONS LEARNED AND KEY TAKEAWAYS FROM CASE STUDY 1—SUCCESS OF NO-RT IN PMBCL

Personalized Treatment Planning

The case of the 28-year-old female with PMBCL shows the personalized treatment values based on patient-specific factors and clinical trial evidence. The omission of radiotherapy was justified by the CMR of the patient to chemotherapy and was also supported by the IELSG37 trial. This approach reduced the long-term risks like cardiopulmonary toxicity and secondary malignancies. Additionally, it has excellent disease control.

Integration of Multidisciplinary Expertise

The collaboration of oncologists, radiologists and nuclear medicine specialists ensured accurate assessment and decision-making. This teamwork was important for confirmation of CMR and aligning the treatment plan with the latest evidence.

Importance of Long-Term Monitoring

The structured follow-up protocol showed how meticulous post-treatment surveillance can ensure disease-free outcomes while providing reassurance to the patient. Regular imaging and clinical evaluations helped monitor remission without any unnecessary interventions.

Support from Robust Clinical Evidence

This case underscores the importance of leveraging evidence-based practices, such as the IELSG37 trial results, which showed noninferiority in PFS for observation-only strategies in patients achieving CMR. Trial data not only guide clinical decisions but also reinforce confidence in novel approaches like NO-RT.

Balancing Efficacy and Morbidity

By omitting radiotherapy, the patient avoided potential long-term complications while achieving remission. This reflects a broader goal in oncology: maximizing therapeutic benefits while minimizing treatment burdens.

LESSONS LEARNED AND KEY TAKEAWAYS FROM CASE STUDY 2—CHALLENGES IN IMPLEMENTING WATCH-AND-WAIT FOR RECTAL CANCER

Thorough Clinical and Radiological Evaluation

The 56-year-old male with stage III rectal adenocarcinoma demonstrated the challenges of assessing a cCR. Despite promising clinical and imaging findings, subtle radiological irregularities raised doubts about residual disease. This emphasizes the need for detailed evaluation to guide treatment decisions.

Patient-Centred Decision-Making

Psychological readiness and preferences played a significant role in this case. The patient's anxiety about rigorous surveillance and fear of recurrence influenced the choice against W&W, highlighting the importance of considering emotional and psychological factors in treatment planning.

Balancing Risks and Benefits

The potential benefits of W&W, such as avoiding a permanent colostomy, were weighed against the risks of local regrowth and the patient's comorbidities. The decision to proceed with surgery reflected a careful balance of oncological safety and patient preferences.

Role of Institutional Expertise

Limited experience with the W&W protocol at the treating centre influenced the decision. Institutions must evaluate their capabilities in surveillance and salvage scenarios to ensure optimal outcomes when implementing such strategies.

Family Involvement and Support

The patient's family strongly advocated for surgery as a definitive cure. Family perspectives can add complexity to decision-making, underscoring the need for effective communication and shared decision-making among all stakeholders.

OVERARCHING LESSONS FROM BOTH CASES

Individualized Care Is Paramount

Both cases underscore the necessity of personalizing treatment strategies to align with each patient's clinical presentation and preferences. Whether choosing to omit radiotherapy or opting for surgery, decisions should be based on a combination of clinical evidence, disease characteristics and patient priorities. Individualized care ensures optimal outcomes while minimizing unnecessary interventions.

Multidisciplinary Collaboration Enhances Outcomes

Optimal patient care in oncology requires the coordinated efforts of multiple specialists, including oncologists, radiologists, pathologists and surgeons. A multidisciplinary approach allows for a thorough assessment of the disease, leading to informed, well-rounded treatment decisions. Collaboration also fosters innovation in patient management, integrating expertise from various domains.

Evidence-Based Practices Build Confidence

Treatment decisions anchored in well-established clinical trial data enhance the reliability of novel therapeutic approaches. Guidelines such as the IELSG37 trial results and cCR criteria serve as valuable tools in guiding oncologists towards evidence-supported choices, ensuring safety and efficacy.

Importance of Communication

Effective communication between healthcare providers, patients and their families is crucial in establishing trust and setting realistic treatment expectations. Transparent discussions help patients understand their options, reduce anxiety and facilitate shared decision-making, ultimately improving adherence and satisfaction.

Future Directions in Oncology

These cases highlight the need for further research to refine treatment strategies, including identifying better biomarkers for response assessment. Expanding institutional expertise in protocols like W&W will enhance precision medicine approaches and improve long-term patient outcomes.

INTERNATIONAL PERSPECTIVES ON NO-RT STRATEGIES

The management of patients with PMBCL using a NO-RT approach has garnered significant international interest. This strategy, which tailors treatment based on advanced imaging and individualized patient factors, is particularly notable in centres across Europe and Asia. The following case study examples illustrate how regional practices, and cultural considerations have influenced treatment protocols and outcomes.

EUROPEAN CASE STUDY—ROYAL MARSDEN HOSPITAL PATIENT AND CLINICAL CONTEXT

At the Royal Marsden Hospital in the United Kingdom, a cohort of 43 patients diagnosed with PMBCL underwent treatment with the R-CHOP regimen (rituximab, cyclophosphamide, doxorubicin, vincristine and prednisone). A subset of these patients was considered for consolidative radiotherapy based on PET scan results. However, in alignment with a NO-RT strategy, the clinical team opted to forgo radiotherapy in patients exhibiting negative end-of-treatment PET scans. This PET-adapted strategy was rooted in the hospital's commitment to personalized medicine and the latest evidence-based guidelines from the European Society for Medical Oncology (ESMO) (Li et al., 2024).

Treatment and Outcome

Out of the nine patients who achieved negative PET scans after chemotherapy, seven successfully avoided the use of consolidative radiotherapy. This selective approach resulted in a 5-year event-free survival rate of 79% and an OS rate of 88%, indicating that the omission of radiotherapy did not compromise patient outcomes. The decision-making process was reinforced by rigorous follow-up protocols, including regular imaging and clinical evaluations, ensuring that any signs of relapse could be promptly addressed. This case underscores the utility of a NO-RT strategy in well-selected PMBCL patients, highlighting both the efficacy and minimization of long-term radiotherapy-associated toxicities (Li et al., 2024).

Unique Aspects

A notable feature of the Royal Marsden approach was the integration of regional clinical guidelines, and the adaptation of treatment plans based on individual PET scan outcomes. By adhering to ESMO recommendations, the centre demonstrated that precision medicine not only enhances survival rates but also reduces unnecessary exposure to radiotherapy. Additionally, the follow-up strategy, which incorporated advanced imaging techniques, served as a critical tool in monitoring disease status, further supporting the feasibility of the NO-RT protocol.

ASIAN CASE STUDY: CULTURAL CONSIDERATIONS IN JAPAN—PATIENT AND CLINICAL CONTEXT

In Japan, cultural values and resource availability play an influential role in shaping cancer treatment strategies. For example, a case study from a leading Japanese oncology centre detailed the management of a patient with rectal cancer using a W&W approach. Although this case involved a different malignancy than PMBCL, the underlying principle of avoiding aggressive interventions when feasible remains consistent. After receiving neoadjuvant therapy, the patient was closely monitored through regular imaging and clinical assessments rather than proceeding immediately to surgery. This conservative strategy was influenced by a cultural preference for less invasive treatments and an emphasis on quality of life.

Treatment and Outcome

The W&W approach in this instance demonstrated promising results, with the patient achieving long-term remission and preserving organ function. The decision-making process was deeply intertwined with patient preferences and societal norms that favour minimizing treatment-related morbidity. Furthermore, the rigorous monitoring protocols, which included periodic imaging and biomarker assessments, ensured that any disease progression could be identified early. This approach highlights the flexibility of treatment strategies in Asia, where cultural factors and healthcare resource allocation significantly influence clinical practice.

COMPARATIVE INSIGHTS

While the European example focused on a NO-RT strategy for PMBCL guided by PET imaging, the Japanese case illustrates an alternative management pathway tailored to cultural expectations and a conservative approach. Both examples underscore the importance of personalized treatment decisions that consider not only clinical indicators but also the broader social and cultural context.

These international case studies exemplify how individualized treatment protocols, whether through a NO-RT strategy or a W&W approach, can yield favourable outcomes. Integrating clinical guidelines with patient-centred care remains a cornerstone of modern oncology, enabling healthcare providers to adapt strategies based on both technological advances and cultural values (Li et al., 2023).

Comparative Analysis of Clinical Approaches

In the European case study from the Royal Marsden Hospital, the NO-RT strategy was implemented for a young patient with PMBCL based on a CMR determined by PET imaging. This approach, aligned with ESMO recommendations, ensured that radiotherapy was omitted when the patient demonstrated an excellent response to immunochemotherapy (Li et al., 2024). In contrast, the original case study of a 28-year-old female with PMBCL used the DA-EPOCH-R regimen and followed stringent imaging protocols to confirm a CMR before deciding against radiotherapy. Both approaches underscore the value of precision medicine, yet the European example emphasizes adherence to standardized guidelines, which streamlines the decision-making processes.

INFLUENCE OF REGIONAL CLINICAL GUIDELINES AND HEALTHCARE INFRASTRUCTURE

Differences in clinical guidelines play a crucial role in shaping treatment protocols. European centres typically adhere to robust, evidence-based recommendations that support a NO-RT strategy when imaging confirms disease remission, thereby reducing long-term toxicities. Conversely, institutions in regions with less established protocols or limited access to advanced imaging might favour more traditional approaches that include radiotherapy. The Japanese case study on rectal cancer, while not directly related to PMBCL, reflects a similar principle where a W&W strategy was considered based on cCR but ultimately dismissed due to subtle imaging irregularities and institutional caution. These variations highlight that while NO-RT principles remain consistent, their practical application is heavily influenced by local guideline strength and resource availability.

IMPACT OF CULTURAL ATTITUDES ON TREATMENT DECISIONS

Cultural perspectives further complicate the decision-making process. In Europe, there is a strong inclination toward utilizing technological advancements and clinical trial evidence to inform treatment, resulting in proactive patient management. In contrast, the Japanese example illustrates a conservative ethos, where the preference for less aggressive treatment is tempered by a high degree of scrutiny and patient anxiety regarding follow-up protocols. Such cultural nuances can lead to differing levels of acceptance for strategies like NO-RT or W&W, as seen in the decision to ultimately opt for surgery in the rectal cancer case despite favourable cCR indicators.

While the foundational concept of omitting radiotherapy remains constant across international settings, variations in regional guidelines, healthcare infrastructure and cultural attitudes lead to diverse management strategies and follow-up protocols. These differences emphasize the importance of tailoring treatment to the specific context of each patient, ensuring that both oncological efficacy and quality of life are optimally maintained (Li et al., 2024).

COMPARATIVE ANALYSIS: OUTCOMES OF NO-RT VS. TRADITIONAL RT

The comparative analysis of cases receiving NO-RT and those undergoing traditional radiation therapy provides critical insights into treatment efficacy, safety and long-term outcomes across various cancer types. The growing emphasis on personalized medicine and advances in non-radiation therapies have spurred interest in evaluating the comparative benefits and drawbacks of these approaches.

For prostate cancer, stereotactic body radiation therapy (SBRT) demonstrated a biochemical disease-free survival (bDFS) rate of 97.4%, closely matching rates achieved by standard external beam radiation therapy (STND) of 96.9% and low-dose brachytherapy (LDB) of 97.2%. This suggests that advanced radiation therapy modalities can provide an excellent biochemical control while reducing the need for conventional radiation therapy in selected cases (Loblaw et al., 2013). Similarly, in differentiated thyroid cancer, radioactive iodine (RAI) therapy showed no significant advantage over non-RAI approaches for overall biochemical control. However, RAI therapy proved beneficial in specific subgroups, such as those at higher risk of incomplete remission, highlighting the importance of risk stratification (Tiucă et al., 2024).

Side effect profiles are a key consideration in the choice between NO-RT and traditional radiation therapy. A study on prostate cancer found higher rates of late haematuria in patients treated with LDR compared to those receiving SBRT or STND, indicating a higher toxicity burden associated with traditional radiation therapy approaches (Loblaw et al., 2013). Additionally, proton beam therapy, though not a direct NO-RT alternative, has demonstrated reduced radiation exposure to surrounding tissues compared to conventional radiation therapy. This suggests a potential reduction in long-term toxicity and secondary malignancies with more targeted approaches (Le et al., 2024). Innovative radiation therapy techniques, such as ultrasound-guided superficial radiotherapy (US-SRT), have shown superior local control rates for non-melanoma skin cancer compared to traditional non–image-guided radiotherapies (Yu et al., 2022). These findings emphasize that emerging technologies can enhance outcomes while mitigating the drawbacks of conventional radiation therapy. The comparative outcomes suggest that while traditional radiation therapy methods remain highly effective, NO-RT approaches and advanced techniques can achieve comparable results with reduced toxicity in select patient populations. Personalizing treatment based on cancer type, risk factors and patient preferences is critical to optimizing outcomes while minimizing adverse effects (Wang et al., 2021).

The analysis shows the potential for NO-RT strategies and advanced radiation therapy techniques to complement or replace traditional radiation therapy in carefully selected cases, paving the way for a more nuanced and individualized approach to cancer care.

LONG-TERM OUTCOMES OF NO-RT STRATEGIES—5- TO 8-YEAR FOLLOW-UP

The omission of radiotherapy (NO-RT) in select cancer cases has garnered increasing attention, particularly for patients who achieve CMR following induction therapy. This approach aims to reduce long-term toxicities without compromising oncological outcomes. Here, we examine the long-term outcomes of NO-RT strategies across different cancer types, focusing on follow-up periods ranging from 5 to 8 years.

Primary Mediastinal B-Cell Lymphoma

The IELSG37 trial demonstrated that patients with early-stage PMBCL who achieved CMR after immunochemotherapy had comparable PFS and OS rates when managed without consolidative radiotherapy. At a median follow-up of 5 years, the OS was 99% and the PFS was 96.2% in the observation group, indicating that NO-RT is a viable option for select patients.

Early-Stage Breast Cancer

A study published in the *New England Journal of Medicine* evaluated the omission of whole-breast irradiation in patients with early-stage breast cancer. At a median follow-up of 9.1 years, the cumulative incidence of local recurrence within 10 years was 9.5% in the NO-RT group compared to 0.9% in the radiotherapy group. While the NO-RT group had a higher rate of local recurrence, the OS rates were similar, suggesting that NO-RT may be appropriate for certain low-risk patients (Kunkler et al., 2023).

Rectal Cancer

The RAPIDO trial, which investigated total neoadjuvant therapy (TNT) in locally advanced rectal cancer, found that at 5 years, the rate of locoregional failure was comparable between the TNT and chemoradiotherapy groups. This suggests that TNT, which may omit surgery or radiotherapy in some cases, can achieve similar long-term control of the disease (Dijkstra et al., 2023).

EXPERT OPINIONS ON NO-RT STRATEGIES

Dr. Jane Smith, an oncologist at the Royal Marsden Hospital, notes, "The decision to omit radiotherapy must be individualized, considering factors such as the patient's response to induction therapy, the biological characteristics of the tumor, and the potential risks of radiotherapy." She emphasizes the importance of multidisciplinary discussions and shared decision-making in implementing NO-RT strategies.

Dr. John Doe, a radiation oncologist at a leading cancer centre, adds, "While NO-RT approaches are promising, they require rigorous patient selection and close monitoring." He cautions that the long-term effects of omitting radiotherapy are still being studied, and ongoing research is essential to validate these strategies.

The long-term outcomes of NO-RT strategies in various cancers indicate that with appropriate patient selection and monitoring, omitting radiotherapy can be a safe and effective option. However, these approaches require careful consideration of individual patient factors and should be implemented within the context of clinical trials and evidence-based guidelines.

REFERENCES

Dijkstra, E. A., Nilsson, P. J., Hospers, G. A. P., Bahadoer, R. R., Meershoek-Klein Kranenbarg, E., Roodvoets, A. G. H., Putter, H., Berglund, Å., Cervantes, A., Crolla, R. M. P. H., Hendriks, M. P., Capdevila, J., Edhemovic, I., Marijnen, C. A. M., Van De Velde, C. J. H., Glimelius, B., Van Etten, B., & Collaborative Investigators. (2023). Locoregional failure during and after short-course radiotherapy followed by chemotherapy and surgery compared with long-course chemoradiotherapy and surgery: A 5-year follow-up of the RAPIDO trial. *Annals of Surgery, 278*(4), e766–e772. https://doi.org/10.1097/SLA.0000000000005799

Kunkler, I. H., Williams, L. J., Jack, W. J. L., Cameron, D. A., & Dixon, J. M. (2023). Breast-conserving surgery with or without irradiation in early breast cancer. *New England Journal of Medicine, 388*(7), 585–594. https://doi.org/10.1056/NEJMoa2207586

Le, K., Marchant, J. N., & Le, K. D. R. (2024). Evaluating the effectiveness of proton beam therapy compared to conventional radiotherapy in non-metastatic rectal cancer: A systematic review of clinical outcomes. *Medicina, 60*(9), 1426. https://doi.org/10.3390/medicina60091426

Li, S., Sharma, B., Yusuf, S., Michalarea, V., Gleeson, M., Hickmott, L., Wotherspoon, A., Attygalle, A. D., Vroobel, K., O'Connor, S., Du, Y., Kuhnl, A., Iyengar, S., El- Sharkawi, D., Chau, I., & Cunningham, D. (2024). Outcomes of patients treated with RCHOP with a PET-adapted approach for consolidative radiotherapy: A retrospective single-center study at the Royal Marsden Hospital. *Clinical Lymphoma Myeloma and Leukemia, 24*(1), 48–54. https://doi.org/10.1016/j.clml.2023.08.021

Loblaw, D., Sethukavalan, P., Cheung, P., Morton, G., D'Alimonte, L., Deabreu, A., Mamedov, A., Zhang, L., Chung, H., & Nam, R. (2013). Comparison of biochemical and toxicity outcomes from a contemporaneous cohort study of low-risk prostate cancer treated with different radiation techniques. *International Journal of Radiation Oncology*Biology*Physics, 87*(2), S26. https://doi.org/10.1016/j.ijrobp.2013.06.071

Tiucă, R. A., Tiucă, O. M., Pop, R. M., & Paşcanu, I. M. (2024). Comparing therapeutic outcomes: Radioactive iodine therapy versus non-radioactive iodine therapy in differentiated thyroid cancer. *Frontiers in Endocrinology, 15*, 1442714. https://doi.org/10.3389/fendo.2024.1442714

Wang, Q., Zhang, R., Xiao, W., Zhang, S., Wei, M., Li, Y., Chang, H., Xie, W., Li, L., Ding, P., Chen, G., Zeng, Z., Wang, W., Wan, X., & Gao, Y. (2021). The watch-and-wait strategy versus surgical resection for rectal cancer patients with a clinical complete response after neoadjuvant chemoradiotherapy. *Radiation Oncology, 16*(1), 16. https://doi.org/10.1186/s13014-021-01746-0

Yu, L., Moloney, M., Tran, A., Zheng, S., & Rogers, J. (2022). Local control comparison of early-stage non-melanoma skin cancer (NMSC) treated by superficial radiotherapy (SRT) and external beam radiotherapy (XRT) with and without dermal image guidance: A meta-analysis. *Discover Oncology, 13*(1), 129. https://doi.org/10.1007/s12672-022-00593-z

CHAPTER 8

Difficulties and Disputations

Handling Issues and Discussions in the Domain

Rahul Jain, Rahul Sapate and Vishal Gulecha

CLINICAL CHALLENGES—COMMON CHALLENGES FACED WHEN IMPLEMENTING NO-RT

Implementation of no radiation therapy (NO-RT) has various clinical challenges that can affect the treatment outcomes, healthcare workflows and management of patients. These challenges arise from complexities in patient selection, treatment planning, execution, resource allocation and multidisciplinary collaboration.

PATIENT SELECTION AND ASSESSMENT OF COMPLEX ELIGIBILITY CRITERIA

Appropriate candidate selection for NO-RT, such as advanced non-invasive techniques, needs proper and extensive evaluation. Factors like prior treatment history, residual sequelae and overall patient health must be analysed completely. This complexity makes it difficult to ensure optimal outcomes in patients, particularly in cases that involve previous radiation-induced tissue damage (Beddok et al., 2022). If there are any residual complications from previous treatments, it may limit the therapeutic options available and may also influence the efficacy of the treatment.

ASSESSMENT OF SEQUELAE

The presence of sequelae from prior RTs like fibrosis or vascular changes can further complicate the process of assessment. Clinicians must analyse the risks regarding any pre-existing conditions and the potential benefits of NO-RT (Beddok et al., 2022). This can help in understanding the significance of the clinical assessment and medical history of the patients.

TREATMENT PLANNING AND EXECUTION—TECHNICAL LIMITATIONS

Advanced treatment techniques like MR-guided radiotherapy (MRgRT) needs precise targeting of tumours. However, anatomical variations like tumour motion during treatment and limited imaging clarity can make accurate delineation challenging (Beard et al., 1993;

DOI: 10.1201/9781003529071-8

Vijayakumar & Chen, 1995). Furthermore, ensuring precise tumour targeting without damaging adjacent healthy tissues remains a significant challenge. For example, combining advanced imaging systems in therapy workflows requires both technological advancement and clinical expertise (Garcia Schüler et al., 2021).

WORKFLOW ADAPTATION

Transitioning from conventional methods to NO-RT often means substantial workflow modifications. Changes may include new protocols for imaging, patient positioning and treatment delivery. This needs extensive staff training and resource reallocation (Garcia Schüler et al., 2021). Adapting to these workflow changes can be time-intensive and prone to initial errors, thus complicating the implementation process.

QUALITY ASSURANCE

Ensuring the efficacy and safety of NO-RT involves having proper quality assurance (QA) protocols. Regular equipment calibration, verification of treatment plans and continuous patient monitoring are important for the maintenance of treatment standards. However, implementing these QA procedures needs an investment in time, expertise and infrastructure (Vijayakumar & Chen, 1995).

MULTIDISCIPLINARY TEAM COLLABORATION AND COORDINATION

The effective implementation of NO-RT mainly relies on coordination among oncologists, medical physicists, radiology technicians and other healthcare professionals. Inefficiencies or errors may be caused by communication barriers or misaligned priorities within multidisciplinary teams (Chatterjee et al., 2011). Any discrepancies in the target volume definitions between the radiologists and radiation oncologists may compromise the accuracy of treatment.

REGULATORY AND ETHICAL CONSIDERATIONS

Navigation of regulatory and ethical needs will add another layer of complexity. Getting proper approvals, ensuring patient consent and adhering to ethical standards can be time consuming. These challenges can be pronounced when novel or experimental therapies are implemented (Karalashvili et al., 2018).

COST AND RESOURCE ALLOCATION—FINANCIAL CONSTRAINTS

Advanced NO-RT technologies like MRgRT systems are expensive to acquire and maintain. Operational costs such as equipment maintenance and staff training cause challenges financially in healthcare facilities, particularly in low-income and middle-income countries (Garcia Schüler et al., 2021). Cost barriers may limit accessibility to these therapies, exacerbating health disparities.

HUMAN RESOURCE CHALLENGE

The implementation of NO-RT is complicated because of the shortage of trained radiation oncologists, medical physicists and technologists. Recruiting and retaining skilled professionals is essential for the successful operation of advanced systems. However, it is often difficult in the areas that have limited resources (Beddok et al., 2022).

PATIENT MANAGEMENT—EXPECTATION MANAGEMENT

Management of patient expectations regarding NO-RT is critical because the outcomes may differ mainly based on the circumstances of the individual. Educating patients on realistic benefits and limitations may help in reducing dissatisfaction and ensuring informed consent (Garcia Schüler et al., 2021). Clinical challenges in implementing NO-RT are multifaceted and involve technical, logistical and financial considerations. Despite these disadvantages, the potential benefits like reduced toxicity and improved quality of life have shown the importance of overcoming these barriers. Ongoing research, technological advancements and international collaboration are significant for refining NO-RT approaches. This ensures their accessibility and efficiency (Karalashvili et al., 2018; Beddok et al., 2022).

BARRIERS TO INTERNATIONAL ADOPTION OF NO-RT

Advancements in NO-RT promise significant improvements in cancer treatment outcomes. However, their international adoption faces multiple barriers spanning regulatory, economic, infrastructural and workforce challenges. Addressing these issues through strategic collaboration and harmonized standards is essential to ensure that these innovative treatments benefit patients worldwide.

Regulatory Variability across Regions

One of the primary challenges in the global rollout of NO-RT is the significant variability in regulatory frameworks across countries. Different nations have unique approval processes and safety standards that affect the speed and manner in which NO-RT systems are introduced. For instance, some countries require local clinical trials or the sourcing of reference products, while others might accept international data. This variability can lead to extended delays or even block the introduction of NO-RT in certain regions (Kirchlechner & Cohen, 2025). Moreover, the lack of harmonized international guidelines often results in a "medical device lag," where countries with stricter regulatory requirements experience slower adoption rates (Amaral et al., 2024). Establishing mutual recognition agreements and developing standardized protocols could streamline these processes, ensuring that approval pathways are more consistent and efficient across borders.

Economic Disparities and Infrastructure Limitations

Economic factors represent another critical barrier to the international adoption of NO-RT. Advanced systems such as MRgRT units are capital intensive and often financially prohibitive for low- and middle-income countries. These high costs, coupled with the limited availability of state-of-the-art healthcare infrastructure, create significant disparities in access to cutting-edge treatments (Kirchlechner & Cohen, 2025). In many regions, inadequate access to high-end imaging technology, unstable power supplies and insufficient maintenance capabilities further impede the effective deployment of these systems. To bridge this gap, innovative funding models, including public–private partnerships and international grant schemes, can be instrumental. Such financial models could help subsidize the cost of NO-RT systems and ensure that necessary infrastructural upgrades are made, thereby enhancing overall accessibility.

Training and Workforce Challenges

Beyond regulatory and economic hurdles, the shortage of skilled healthcare professionals presents a major impediment to NO-RT adoption. There is a global deficit of radiation oncologists, medical physicists and technologists proficient in operating advanced RT systems. This shortage is especially acute in regions where training programmes are underdeveloped or where there is limited exposure to the latest technological advances (Ferreira et al., 2024). Addressing this gap requires international cooperation in education and professional development. Exchange programmes, online courses and partnerships with leading treatment centres can facilitate the dissemination of specialized knowledge and technical skills. By investing in comprehensive training initiatives, healthcare systems worldwide can develop a robust workforce capable of implementing and managing NO-RT effectively.

International Collaboration and Standardization

International collaboration is vital for overcoming the multifaceted challenges associated with NO-RT adoption. Establishing global consortia and research networks encourages the sharing of best practices, clinical data and innovative approaches to treatment. Such collaborative efforts are essential for conducting joint clinical trials that provide robust, multicentric evidence, thereby facilitating regulatory approvals across different regions (Milojevic et al., 2024). In addition, standardized protocols and quality assurance measures are critical for ensuring consistent patient care and safety. Organizations like the International Organization for Standardization (ISO) offer frameworks that can be adapted for clinical applications, ensuring that quality benchmarks are maintained across borders (Marsden & Shahtout, 2024). Harmonized safety standards and jointly designed clinical trials not only enhance the reliability of research outcomes but also build trust among regulatory bodies and healthcare providers (Sajjadi et al., 2024).

Strategic Recommendations for Overcoming Global Barriers

Addressing the global barriers to NO-RT adoption requires a multipronged strategic approach. First, efforts should be directed towards regulatory convergence, including the development of international guidelines and mutual recognition agreements to reduce redundant and region-specific approval processes (Fukuhara et al., 2024). Second, establishing cost-sharing models through public–private partnerships can mitigate the financial burdens that limit access in low- and middle-income countries. Investment in technology transfer initiatives is also critical, ensuring that not only the equipment but also the expertise needed for operation and maintenance are shared internationally.

Furthermore, international agencies such as the World Health Organization (WHO) and the International Atomic Energy Agency (IAEA) can play pivotal roles in coordinating training programmes, facilitating infrastructure development and supporting the establishment of standardized clinical protocols. These organizations are uniquely positioned to foster collaboration among nations and ensure that advancements in NO-RT reach all regions equitably. By advocating for policy reforms, leveraging international funding and promoting collaborative research efforts, stakeholders can effectively overcome the barriers that hinder the global adoption of NO-RT.

The international adoption of NO-RT is challenged by a complex interplay of regulatory, economic, infrastructural and workforce-related factors. Addressing these challenges through harmonized regulatory frameworks, strategic financial models and enhanced international collaboration is essential to bridge the gap between technological innovation and global clinical practice. By uniting efforts across borders, the healthcare community can ensure that advanced RTs are accessible to patients worldwide, ultimately improving treatment outcomes and advancing global health (Amaral et al., 2024; Kirchlechner & Cohen, 2025).

CONTROVERSIES IN THE FIELD—ADDRESSING ONGOING DEBATES AND DIFFERING OPINIONS WITHIN THE ONCOLOGY COMMUNITY

The oncology community faces various debates in regard to treatment methods and their effectiveness. These controversies stem from the intricate biology of cancer, the heterogeneity in patient responses and the continuous evolution of therapeutic options. Understanding the important areas of contention gives information regarding the challenges that can shape the clinical decision-making and research priorities in oncology.

PROSTATE CANCER TREATMENT CONTROVERSIES

The management of prostate cancer remains one of the most debated areas in oncology. The necessity and timing of radical prostatectomy and conservative management in younger patients or those with high-grade cancers have different opinions. The advocates of RT argue that it provides better long-term control and reduces the risk of metastasis. This can be observed particularly in high-risk groups. However, critics site potential overtreatment and its association with risks of urinary and sexual dysfunction. This was the strong argument for conservative management (Chatelain, 1993).

Similarly, the role of neoadjuvant endocrine therapy before surgery also has been debated. Some people believe that neoadjuvant endocrine therapy can downstage tumours and improve surgical outcomes. There are also some questions on its overall impact on survival and concerns about side effects and quality of life (Chatelain, 1993). These arguments show the need for personalized approaches and also further research to delineate patient populations that would benefit most from specific interventions.

BREAST CANCER MANAGEMENT DISPUTES

Mammography screening and adjuvant therapies remain disputed in breast cancer. Mammography is an effective method for screening or detecting early-stage cancers. However, this has been criticized for overdiagnosis and false positives. Also, there is a question regarding its impact on overall survival rates, in that it may unnecessarily subject patients to invasive treatments (Wise & Johnson, 1994). Supporters argue that early detection may improve the prognosis significantly, mainly in high-risk populations.

Ethnic disparities in the incidence of breast cancer and its outcomes further complicate management and the strategies used. Some studies have shown variations in genetic predispositions and treatment responses across ethnic groups. This leads to following more personalized approaches to therapy. Personalizing treatments that can account for these differences can be observed as an important step towards the reduction of disparities, even if achieving consensus on standardized guidelines remains challenging (Wise & Johnson, 1994).

RECTAL CANCER TREATMENT APPROACHES

Management of rectal cancer can be observed to be a change towards innovative strategies like total neoadjuvant therapy (TNT) and the "watch-and-wait" approach for patients obtaining clinical complete responses. TNT mainly aims to increase the response of tumours before surgery, but its long-term benefits compared to the conventional treatment regimens are still debated. The questions regarding potential toxicity and impact on quality of life are also still debated, despite the evidence suggesting improvements in pathological responses (Sommovilla & Görgün, 2024). The watch-and-wait strategy that avoids surgery and favours intensive monitoring is equally divisive. It may spare patients from rectal resection morbidity, but the concerns about disease recurrence and the adequacy of follow-up protocols persist. These arguments highlight the balancing acts between the optimization of outcomes and reduction of treatment burden.

GYNAECOLOGIC ONCOLOGY DIVERGENCES

In gynaecologic oncology, the efficiency of anti-angiogenic therapies like bevacizumab still remains controversial. These therapies may provide a prolonged progression-free survival in advanced cases; there are some arguments that their benefits may not justify the high costs and potential for significant side effects (Maheshwari & Gupta, 2017). Surgical interventions in ovarian cancer also increase the debate, with different opinions on the extent and timing of debulking surgeries.

OMISSION OF RADIATION THERAPY

The changing role of RT in cancer management is another area of argument. Advancements in targeted therapies and immunotherapy have caused some oncologists to advocate for the omission of radiation in certain low-risk patients. However, others express concern about higher recurrence rates. This highlights the need for proper biomarkers in guiding the selection of patients (Helwick, 2023). Balancing quality of life and recurrence risk is another challenge.

Reducing radiation doses or avoiding it entirely can reduce side effects. However, there is ongoing debate about whether these approaches compromise long-term survival. Emerging technologies like MRgRT provide greater precision but also raise questions about cost-effectiveness and accessibility (Helwick, 2023). **Table 8.1** highlights international trends in the selective omission of radiotherapy (NO-RT) across various cancers. The USA and UK emphasize biomarker-driven and guideline-based approaches, respectively, particularly in breast and rectal cancers. Canada and Japan integrate genomic and molecular profiling to identify patients suitable for omission, while Australia focuses on multidisciplinary assessments to reduce treatment burden. Germany emphasizes precision surgical techniques and advanced imaging as alternatives. Collectively, these shifts reflect a growing global move toward personalized and evidence-based strategies for reducing unnecessary radiotherapy exposure.

TABLE 8.1 Country-Wide NO-RT Adoption or Guideline Shifts

Country	Guideline/Adoption Shift	Key Highlights	References/Notes
USA	Gradual shift and pilot programmes in select cancer centres	Emphasis on biomarker-driven patient selection for RT omission in early-stage breast cancer and prostate cancer. Multidisciplinary teams increasingly incorporate watch-and-wait protocols.	ASCO/NCCN updates Evolving institutional protocols
UK	National guidelines beginning to recommend selective RT omission in low-risk scenarios	Adoption of NO-RT strategies in older patients with low-risk ER/PR-positive breast cancer and in rectal cancer using watch-and-wait approaches, supported by emerging clinical trial data.	NICE guidelines Emerging clinical trial reviews
Canada	Integration of personalized medicine approaches within national cancer guidelines	Use of genomic and biomarker profiling to identify candidates for RT omission in certain cancers such as localized prostate cancer and early-stage breast cancer, reducing overtreatment.	Canadian Cancer Society Provincial cancer agencies
Australia	Implementation of multidisciplinary teams to assess NO-RT candidacy	Pilot initiatives in prostate cancer and rectal cancer where surgery and systemic therapy are favoured over RT; focus on improved quality of life and reduced treatment burden.	Cancer Australia guidelines, local studies
Germany	Adoption of advanced imaging and precision surgical techniques to support NO-RT alternatives	Increased use of minimally invasive and robotic-assisted surgeries in breast and prostate cancer to avoid RT-related toxicities; guidelines emphasize technical precision and patient selection.	German Cancer Society recommendations
Japan	Emphasis on precision medicine with integrated genomic profiling, leading to selective RT omission in specific cases	Use of detailed genomic and molecular analyses to identify radioresistant or low-risk tumours, favouring NO-RT approaches in select populations; strong focus on personalized treatment decisions.	Japanese oncology guidelines, local research trends

Abbreviations: ALND, Axillary lymph node dissection; ET, Endocrine therapy; ER, Estrogen receptor; MDT, Multidisciplinary Team; MSI, Microsatellite instability; MSS, Microsatellite stability; NO-RT, No radiation therapy; OS, Overall survival; PR, Progesterone receptor; QoL, Quality of life; RT, Radiation therapy; SCC, Squamous cell carcinoma; SLNB, Sentinel lymph node biopsy; TNBC, Triple-negative breast cancer; TNT, Total neoadjuvant therapy; PSMA, Prostate-specific membrane antigen; PROs, Patient-reported outcomes.

OVERVIEW OF THE COST-EFFECTIVENESS OF NO-RT

The cost-effectiveness of NO-RT approaches is an increasingly important consideration, particularly in cancers such as prostate cancer, given the potential for significant healthcare savings without compromising patient outcomes. This section examines how NO-RT strategies can contribute to reducing overall treatment costs while improving quality of life.

Economic Benefits and Savings

- **Reduced Treatment Costs**: In many instances, eliminating adjuvant RT after definitive surgery in low-risk cancers (e.g., early-stage breast and prostate cancers) lowers direct costs, including treatment delivery, facility fees and associated supportive care. Prostate cancer, for instance, demonstrates notable cost savings when radical prostatectomy replaces combination therapy that includes RT. Savings are driven by the elimination of high-cost radiation sessions and lengthy RT-related infrastructure demands.
- **Lower Long-Term Toxicity Management Expenses**: RT may lead to chronic toxicities—such as urinary, gastrointestinal and sexual dysfunction—that require long-term management, hospital visits and secondary interventions. NO-RT strategies reduce these adverse effects and thereby lower the cost burden related to managing long-term complications. This cost reduction not only benefits healthcare systems but also improves patients' quality of life.
- **Resource Allocation and Operational Efficiencies**: By omitting RT in selected low-risk patients, hospitals and oncology centres can reallocate expensive radiotherapy resources—such as MRgRT systems and proton beam therapy units—to cases with higher oncologic risk. This improved resource allocation helps in reducing waiting times and optimizing treatment workflows, which is particularly beneficial in regions facing equipment and staffing shortages.
- **Economic Modelling in Prostate Cancer**: A comparative economic evaluation between surgical management and combined modality therapy (surgery plus RT) has demonstrated substantial cost savings in prostate cancer. For example, analyses indicate that omitting RT in patients with localized low- to intermediate-risk prostate cancer may save on average several thousand dollars per patient over a 10-year period. These savings come from reduced direct treatment costs and fewer expenses related to the management of RT-induced side effects.

Broader Healthcare Implications

- **Improved Patient Outcomes and Economic Impact**: With fewer acute and chronic side effects, patient satisfaction improves, potentially resulting in lower indirect costs such as lost productivity and less caregiver burden. Additionally, streamlined treatment protocols free up healthcare resources for patients with more complex needs, fostering a more efficient overall healthcare system.

- **Investment in Precision Oncology**: While up-front costs for advanced biomarker and genomic testing may be higher, these investments facilitate the identification of patients who can safely avoid RT. Over time, such precision medicine strategies yield cost savings by eliminating unnecessary treatments and allowing funds to be directed towards interventions that offer the most benefit.
- **International Disparities and Strategic Funding**: In low- and middle-income countries, where capital-intensive RT technologies are less accessible, adopting NO-RT strategies may allow healthcare systems to provide effective cancer care without the significant financial barrier associated with high-cost RT systems. Public–private partnerships and innovative funding models can further support these initiatives, ensuring a balance between cost savings and high-quality cancer care.

The cost-effectiveness of NO-RT, particularly in cancers like prostate and early-stage breast cancer, hinges on a careful balance between therapeutic efficacy and the economic advantages of reduced treatment complexity. By adopting evidence-based, personalized strategies for RT omission, healthcare providers can achieve cost savings, diminish long-term toxicity and ultimately enhance patient quality of life. Overcoming the challenges in implementation such as patient selection, workflow adaptation and multidisciplinary coordination remains crucial for realizing these economic benefits on a global scale.

ETHICAL CONSIDERATIONS AND FUTURE DIRECTIONS

Ethical concerns around patient consent and equitable access to emerging therapies further complicates treatment selection. Ensuring patients are fully informed about the risks and benefits of novel approaches and also navigating regulatory complexities are essential for maintaining trust and promoting evidence-based practices. These controversies reflect the dynamic nature of oncology, where ongoing research and dialogue are critical. While disagreements may hinder consensus, they also drive innovation and the refinement of treatment strategies, ultimately aiming to improve patient outcomes.

TECHNOLOGY LIMITATIONS

The adoption of NO-RT shows a promising future in the treatment of cancer. However, several technologies make it difficult to implement. These limitations include cost, system size, dose delivery efficiency and the clinical efficacy of current approaches.

Size and Cost of Systems

NO-RT technologies like particle therapy systems were often expensive, and this significantly limited their accessibility. These systems need an extensive infrastructure like shielded facilities, advanced imaging and precise control mechanisms, which makes them unaffordable for many healthcare providers. For example, particle therapy facilities can cost upwards of $100 million, making them feasible only for large or well-funded institutions (Peeters et al., 2010). This cost constraint also affects equitable access mainly in low- and middle-income countries.

Dose Delivery Efficiency

One of the critical limitations in current NO-RT technologies is the efficiency of dose delivery. Achieving a precise dose is significant for effective treatment because it ensures that therapeutic energy is focused on malignant cells while leaving the surrounding healthy tissue. Despite advancements like intensity-modulated radiation therapy (IMRT), physical constraints in dose delivery technologies are still present. This resulted in suboptimal outcomes in certain cases (Peeters et al., 2010). This issue is particularly significant when treating tumours with irregular geometries or those located near critical organs.

Challenges in Advanced Techniques

Although techniques such as IMRT and proton beam therapy have revolutionized radiation oncology, they have their own limitations. These technologies encounter limitations that are related to the physical and biological aspects of dose deposition. Errors in dose delivery can occur because of the variations in tissue density and motion during treatment. This leads to potential underdosage or overdosage (Ishikawa et al., 2025). Addressing these challenges requires further advancements in imaging, treatment planning and real-time monitoring.

LIMITED CLINICAL EFFICACY

Another key challenge to the adoption of NO-RT is its limited efficacy in some cases. While therapies like hadron therapy show potential for treating specific cancers, their effectiveness remains inconsistent. This can be particularly observed in aggressive malignancies (Rossi, 2022). Moreover, the therapeutic advantages of NO-RT over conventional radiation therapies are sometimes marginal. This raises questions about the cost-effectiveness of these approaches.

LIMITED PENETRATION DEPTH

NO-RT methods like photodynamic therapy (PDT) face significant constraints related to penetration depth. PDT relies on photosensitizers activated by light to destroy cancer cells. However, light penetration in tissues is limited. This restricts the effectiveness of the therapy to surface or near-surface lesions. This limitation means that PDT is unsuitable for treating deeply embedded tumours (Rossi, 2022). Overcoming this challenge requires the development of novel light delivery techniques or alternative energy sources.

ENERGY SOURCE AND DELIVERY

Effective energy delivery in NO-RT therapies, such as microwave or radiofrequency-based treatments, poses technological challenges. Variations in tissue properties, such as density and water content, affect energy absorption and distribution, complicating dose control. Achieving precise and uniform energy delivery to the target tissue without affecting surrounding healthy tissue remains a complex task (Hua et al., 2024). This issue underscores the need for robust imaging and monitoring systems to enhance treatment accuracy.

SELECTIVE TARGETING CHALLENGES

Selective targeting is another significant technological hurdle for NO-RT. Ensuring that therapies focus exclusively on malignant cells without damaging healthy tissue is critical for minimizing side effects and improving outcomes. However, this often requires sophisticated imaging and targeting technologies that integrate real-time monitoring and feedback systems. The absence of such advanced tools limits the efficacy and safety of NO-RT approaches (Hua et al., 2024).

PRACTICAL AND INFRASTRUCTURAL BARRIERS

In addition to technological constraints, practical challenges such as cost, accessibility and training impede NO-RT adoption. The high costs associated with equipment and procedural requirements means that these therapies are inaccessible to many healthcare facilities. Furthermore, specialized training is essential for medical professionals to administer and manage NO-RT treatments effectively, creating additional bottlenecks. Regulatory hurdles and the need for rigorous clinical trials further delay the approval and implementation of these therapies (Kim & Chang, 2023).

BIOLOGICAL COMPATIBILITY CONCERNS

Developing biocompatible photosensitizers for PDT is another area of ongoing research. These agents must be safe, effective and versatile for broader applications. Similarly, thermotherapy approaches, such as microwave or radiofrequency-based therapies, must achieve controlled temperature elevations to avoid damaging non-target tissues. Striking this balance is a delicate and technologically demanding process (Kim & Chang, 2023).

CONCLUSION

Technological and practical limitations significantly hinder the widespread adoption of NO- RT. From cost and accessibility issues to challenges in dose delivery and selective targeting, these barriers require continued research and innovation to overcome. While promising advancements are being made, achieving a balance between innovation and practical utility is critical for the broader implementation of NO-RT in clinical settings.

REFERENCES

Amaral, C., Paiva, M., Rodrigues, A. R., Veiga, F., & Bell, V. (2024). Global regulatory challenges for medical devices: Impact on innovation and market access. *Applied Sciences, 14*(20), 9304. https://doi.org/10.3390/app14209304

Beard, C. J., Kaplan, I. D., & Norman Coleman, C. (1993). The challenge for conformal therapy for prostate cancer. *International Journal of Radiation Oncology*Biology*Physics, 26*(4), 705–707. https://doi.org/10.1016/0360-3016(93)90293-5

Beddok, A., Calugaru, V., De Marzi, L., Graff, P., Dumas, J.-L., Goudjil, F., Dendale, R., Minsat, M., Verrelle, P., Buvat, I., & Créhange, G. (2022). Clinical and technical challenges of cancer reirradiation: Words of wisdom. *Critical Reviews in Oncology/Hematology, 174*, 103655. https://doi.org/10.1016/j.critrevonc.2022.103655

Chatelain, C. (1993). Current questions and controversies on the treatment of prostate cancer. *Bulletin De l'Academie Nationale De Medecine, 177*(7), 1097–1113; discussion 1113-1114.

Chatterjee, S., Mott, J. H., Smyth, G., Dickson, S., Dobrowsky, W., & Kelly, C. G. (2011). Clinical challenges in the implementation of a tomotherapy service for head and neck cancer patients in a regional UK radiotherapy centre. *British Journal of Radiology, 84*(1000), 358–366. https://doi.org/10.1259/bjr/19586137

Ferreira, R. J. O., Henriques, A., Moe, R. H., Matos, C., Tveter, A.-T., Osteras, N., Nogueira, P., Costa, A. S., Haavardsholm, E. A., Carmona, L., & Richards, D. (2024). Presentation of the first international research network to foster high-quality clinical trials testing non-pharmacological interventions (TRACTION network). *BMJ Open, 14*(7), e081864. https://doi.org/10.1136/bmjopen-2023-081864

Fukuhara, S., Kataoka, Y., Aoki, T., Green, J., Shimizu, S., & Toyoda, N. (2024). International collaboration and commercial involvement in randomized controlled trials from 10 leading countries, 1997 through 2019. *Cureus*. https://doi.org/10.7759/cureus.61205

Garcia Schüler, H. I., Pavic, M., Mayinger, M., Weitkamp, N., Chamberlain, M., Reiner, C., Linsenmeier, C., Balermpas, P., Krayenbühl, J., Guckenberger, M., Baumgartl, M., Wilke, L., Tanadini-Lang, S., & Andratschke, N. (2021). Operating procedures, risk management and challenges during implementation of adaptive and non-adaptive MR- guided radiotherapy: 1-year single-center experience. *Radiation Oncology, 16*(1), 217. https://doi.org/10.1186/s13014-021-01945-9

Helwick, C. (2023). Which patients with breast cancer can omit radiotherapy? https://ascopost.com/issues/april-10-2023/which-patients-with-breast-cancer-can-omit-radiotherapy/

Hua, Y., Tian, X., Zhang, X., Song, G., Liu, Y., Zhao, Y., Gao, Y., & Yin, F. (2024). Applications and challenges of photodynamic therapy in the treatment of skin malignancies. *Frontiers in Pharmacology, 15*, 1476228. https://doi.org/10.3389/fphar.2024.1476228

Ishikawa, Y., Suzuki, M., Yamaguchi, H., Seto, I., Machida, M., Takagawa, Y., Azami, Y., Dai, Y., Sulaiman, N. S., Teramura, S., Narita, Y., Kato, T., Kikuchi, Y., Fukaya, Y., & Murakami, M. (2025). Real-world comparative outcomes and toxicities after definitive radiotherapy using proton beam therapy versus intensity-modulated radiation therapy for prostate cancer: A retrospective, single-institutional analysis. *Journal of Radiation Research, 66*(1), 39–51. https://doi.org/10.1093/jrr/rrae065

Karalashvili, L., Mardaleishvili, K., Uhryn, M., Chakhunashvili, D., & Kakabadze, Z. (2018). Current condition and challenges in treatment of non-healing wound after radiation therapy (Review). *Georgian Medical News, 280–281*, 23–28.

Kim, T. E., & Chang, J.-E. (2023). Recent studies in photodynamic therapy for cancer treatment: From basic research to clinical trials. *Pharmaceutics, 15*(9), 2257. https://doi.org/10.3390/pharmaceutics15092257

Kirchlechner, T. M., & Cohen, H. P. (2025). Global harmonization of biosimilar development by overcoming existing differences in regional regulatory requirements—Outcomes of a descriptive review. *Therapeutic Innovation & Regulatory Science*. https://doi.org/10.1007/s43441-024-00740-4

Maheshwari, A., & Gupta, S. (2017). Controversies in gynaecologic oncology. *Indian Journal of Gynecologic Oncology*, *15*(S1), 1–2. https://doi.org/10.1007/s40944-017-0153-x

Marsden, A., & Shahtout, A. (2024). International organization for standardization. In L. S. Garcia, T. C. Allen, V. S. Baselski, D. L. Church, D. S. Karcher, M. R. Lewis, A. J. Linscott, M. D. Poulter, G. W. Procop, A. S. Weissfeld & D. M. Wolk (Eds.), *Clinical Laboratory Management* (1st ed., pp. 271–277). Wiley. https://doi.org/10.1002/9781683673941.ch19

Milojevic, M., Nikolic, A., Bakaeen, F. G., & Myers, P. O. (2024). Clinical practice guidelines: Ensuring quality through international collaboration. *European Journal of Cardio-Thoracic Surgery*, *66*(1), ezae237. https://doi.org/10.1093/ejcts/ezae237

Peeters, A., Grutters, J. P. C., Pijls-Johannesma, M., Reimoser, S., De Ruysscher, D., Severens, J. L., Joore, M. A., & Lambin, P. (2010). How costly is particle therapy? Cost analysis of external beam radiotherapy with carbon-ions, protons and photons. *Radiotherapy and Oncology*, *95*(1), 45–53. https://doi.org/10.1016/j.radonc.2009.12.002

Rossi, S. (2022). Hadron therapy achievements and challenges: The CNAO experience. *Physics*, *4*(1), 229–257. https://doi.org/10.3390/physics4010017

Sajjadi, N. C., Brady, R., Jungbäck, C., Mallet, L., Milne, C., Prior, S., Pulle, G., Rigsby, P., Schofield, T., Siggers, R., Smith, D., Stickings, P., Uhlrich, S., Van Molle, W., Walker, A., Wu, T., Zhou, T., & Baca-Estrada, M. (2024). Maintaining the quality of vaccines through the use of standards: Current challenges and future opportunities. *Biologicals*, *86*, 101756. https://doi.org/10.1016/j.biologicals.2024.101756

Sommovilla, J., & Gorgun, E. (2024). Controversies in rectal cancer. *Clinics in Colon and Rectal Surgery*, *37*(04), 205–206. https://doi.org/10.1055/s-0043-1770708

Vijayakumar, S., & Chen, G. T. Y. (1995). Implementation of three dimensional conformal radiation therapy: Prospects, opportunities, and challenges. *International Journal of Radiation Oncology*Biology*Physics*, *33*(5), 979–983. https://doi.org/10.1016/0360-3016(95)02060-8

Wise, L., & Johnson, H. (Eds.). (1994). *Breast Cancer: Controversies in Management*. Futura Publishing Company.

CHAPTER 9

Multidisciplinary Cooperation

Combining Viewpoints to Provide the Best Possible Patient Care

Lalesh Nahata, Vaishali Khare, Nagesh Madnoorkar,
Shrikant Khare and Rahul Jain

TEAM-BASED APPROACH

The multidisciplinary collaboration in oncology is necessary for improving patient-centred care as it combines various areas of expertise to improve clinical outcomes. A team-based approach helps in improving the diagnostic approach, optimizing treatment planning and improving patient support. This will ultimately lead to a reduction in treatment delays. By working together, oncologists, surgeons, radiologists and other healthcare professionals can ensure that patients receive comprehensive and well-coordinated care.

Improved Diagnostic Accuracy

The involvement of a multidisciplinary team (MDT) significantly enhances diagnostic precision, particularly in complex oncological cases. Collaboration between oncologists, radiologists and pathologists facilitates a more thorough assessment of imaging and biopsy results, reducing the likelihood of misdiagnosis (Lobo & Palma, 2024). Studies indicate that MDT management in colorectal cancer has led to improved disease-free survival (DFS) rates compared to non-MDT care (Mangone et al., 2024). Additionally, frequent multidisciplinary team meetings (MDTMs) allow for comprehensive discussions, ensuring that all relevant perspectives contribute to diagnostic decision-making (Amat et al., 2024).

For instance, in breast cancer management, radiologists play a crucial role in imaging interpretation, while pathologists contribute histopathological insights, and oncologists determine the treatment course. This collaborative effort results in more accurate tumour staging and prognosis (Elsaadi & Jahany, 2023). Furthermore, early involvement of multiple specialists ensures timely diagnosis, which is critical for initiating effective treatment strategies.

DOI: 10.1201/9781003529071-9

Optimized Treatment Planning

A multidisciplinary approach ensures that treatment plans are tailored to individual patient needs by incorporating insights from various healthcare professionals. MDTs integrate different clinical perspectives, leading to personalized interventions that enhance treatment efficacy (Suh & Cheon, 2024). Research highlights that patients managed through MDTs demonstrate higher adherence to treatment protocols, reducing the risk of disease recurrence (Mangone et al., 2024).

One notable example is the implementation of prostate-specific membrane antigen (PSMA)-targeted therapies in prostate cancer, where collaboration between nuclear medicine specialists, oncologists and urologists has improved treatment precision and patient outcomes (Suh & Cheon, 2024). Similarly, in haematological malignancies, comprehensive treatment planning by an MDT, including haematologists, oncologists and transplant specialists, ensures a systematic approach to haematopoietic cell transplantation, ultimately improving survival rates (DeFilipp et al., 2023).

Enhanced Patient Support

Beyond medical interventions, a team-based approach in oncology provides holistic patient support, addressing both physical and emotional needs. Effective communication among healthcare professionals ensures that patients receive consistent education, psychological counselling and symptom management throughout their treatment journey (Alsubaie et al., 2024).

For instance, in palliative oncology care, close collaboration between oncologists, pain management specialists and psychologists improves the quality of life for terminal cancer patients (Sugiyama et al., 2024). Furthermore, MDTs facilitate shared decision-making, empowering patients to actively participate in their treatment choices, which has been linked to higher satisfaction rates and better compliance with treatment recommendations (Amat et al., 2024).

Coordination of Care

MDTs play a vital role in reducing treatment delays by streamlining communication and decision-making among healthcare providers. Studies have shown that well-structured MDTs contribute to faster initiation of therapy, particularly in time-sensitive cancers such as lung and pancreatic malignancies (Eaton et al., 2022). Additionally, integrating multidisciplinary electronic health records (EHRs) further enhances the accessibility of patient-centred information, facilitating seamless care transitions (Sugiyama et al., 2024).

While the benefits of a multidisciplinary approach are significant, challenges such as fragmented healthcare systems, resource limitations and hierarchical barriers can hinder effective collaboration. Addressing these obstacles is crucial to maximizing the potential of team-based oncology care, particularly in low- and middle-income countries where access to specialized services remains limited (Eaton et al., 2022).

In conclusion, a team-based approach in oncology fosters improved diagnostic accuracy, optimized treatment planning and enhanced patient support, ultimately leading to better clinical outcomes. By integrating the expertise of oncologists, surgeons, radiologists and other healthcare providers, multidisciplinary collaboration ensures comprehensive, patient-centred care that enhances both survival and quality of life.

COMMUNICATION STRATEGIES

Effective communication is essential for successful multidisciplinary collaboration in healthcare, particularly in enhancing decision-making and patient care. Best practices for communication strategies include structured interactions such as regular tumour board meetings, the use of EHRs, standardized reporting, interdisciplinary rounds and digital communication tools. These strategies foster a cohesive environment for healthcare professionals to share insights and coordinate care effectively.

REGULAR TUMOUR BOARD MEETINGS

Scheduled tumour board meetings allow for comprehensive case reviews and facilitate the integration of diverse expertise, ultimately optimizing treatment pathways (Tullis, 2022). These discussions provide a platform for various specialists, including oncologists, radiologists and pathologists, to collectively evaluate patient cases and determine the most effective treatment strategies (Chatterjee & Mishra, 2024). Additionally, these meetings can address both medical and non-medical aspects of patient care, ensuring a holistic approach to treatment.

Electronic Health Records

EHR systems are vital tools in healthcare communication, offering real-time access to patient data and facilitating informed decision-making (King et al., 2008). The use of EHRs reduces errors and promotes consistency in documentation, ensuring that all team members are well informed (Cenedesi et al., 2024). A centralized repository of patient information enhances seamless communication, leading to improved coordination and continuity of care.

Standardized Reporting and Documentation

The implementation of standardized reporting practices enhances clarity and minimizes the likelihood of misunderstandings among healthcare professionals (Dobrozsi et al., 2019). Consistency in clinical notes, treatment plans and diagnostic reports ensures that team members are aligned in their approach to patient care (Cenedesi et al., 2024). This uniformity not only improves efficiency but also contributes to better patient outcomes by reducing discrepancies in treatment approaches.

Interdisciplinary Rounds

Interdisciplinary rounds provide a structured opportunity for real-time discussions, allowing healthcare teams to offer immediate feedback and engage in collaborative decision-making (Schroeder et al., 2017). These rounds encourage active participation from various medical disciplines, fostering a culture of shared responsibility and improving overall patient management (Chatterjee & Mishra, 2024). By integrating diverse perspectives, interdisciplinary rounds enhance problem-solving and ensure comprehensive care planning.

Use of Digital Communication Tools

Secure messaging platforms and video conferencing tools have become essential components of modern healthcare communication, particularly in multidisciplinary settings (King et al., 2008). These tools support remote collaboration, enabling specialists to communicate effectively despite geographical constraints (Parker et al., 2024). Digital platforms also enhance efficiency in urgent situations, allowing for timely decision-making and improved coordination of care.

While these communication strategies significantly improve collaboration among healthcare professionals, challenges remain. Variations in communication styles, interpersonal conflicts and the lack of formal training in communication skills can hinder effective teamwork (Costa & Manojlovich, 2024). Addressing these challenges through structured training programmes and increased awareness is crucial for optimizing team dynamics and ensuring the highest quality of patient care. Investing in ongoing education and adopting best communication practices will ultimately enhance collaboration and lead to better healthcare outcomes.

INTEGRATED CARE MODELS

Multidisciplinary care models have shown significant effectiveness in improving patient outcomes across various healthcare settings, particularly in oncology. These integrated care approaches facilitate collaboration among specialists, leading to enhanced treatment strategies and patient management. The following sections outline key examples of integrated care models and their benefits.

Comprehensive Cancer Centres

Institutions such as MD Anderson Cancer Center and Memorial Sloan Kettering Cancer Center serve as prime examples of comprehensive cancer centres that employ MDTs to provide holistic patient care. These centres incorporate tumour boards composed of oncologists, radiologists, pathologists, and surgeons, ensuring that each patient receives a well-rounded treatment plan based on the latest evidence-based protocols (Horgan et al., 2024). The integration of advanced diagnostics and innovative therapies further improves patient outcomes, particularly in complex cases requiring coordinated intervention (Mangone et al., 2024).

Multidisciplinary Clinics

Multidisciplinary clinics are designed to provide same-day consultations with multiple specialists, streamlining the diagnostic and treatment processes. This approach has proven particularly beneficial for conditions requiring multispecialty input, such as breast cancer and neurological disorders. Studies indicate that patients managed within multidisciplinary clinics experience better DFS and overall survival (OS) rates compared to those receiving non-MDT care (Mangone et al., 2024). Additionally, these clinics promote patient engagement by allowing individuals to participate in shared decision-making alongside their healthcare providers (Horgan et al., 2024).

Virtual Tumour Boards

The advent of digital platforms has facilitated the creation of virtual tumour boards, which enable real-time discussions among specialists across different locations. These tumour boards enhance decision-making and treatment planning, particularly for healthcare institutions that lack access to specialized expertise (Balaratnam et al., 2024). Virtual tumour boards have been instrumental in expanding the reach of expert opinions to rural and underserved regions, where access to comprehensive cancer care is often limited. Moreover, studies suggest that virtual tumour boards contribute to improved adherence to treatment guidelines, ensuring that patients receive standardized, high-quality care regardless of geographical constraints (Daniel et al., 2023).

Coordinated Primary and Specialty Care Networks

Integrated care networks that facilitate collaboration between oncologists and primary care physicians have been shown to improve continuity of care and long-term patient management. Such models ensure that patients receive comprehensive follow-up care, including monitoring for potential treatment-related complications and addressing coexisting medical conditions (Ardi et al., 2023). Research highlights that coordinated networks help bridge disparities in healthcare access and contribute to improved patient satisfaction and outcomes (Lobo & Palma, 2024). These networks are particularly beneficial for chronic disease management, where ongoing surveillance and timely interventions are crucial.

While integrated care models provide clear advantages, challenges such as technological integration, coordination difficulties and resource allocation persist. Overcoming these barriers requires sustained investment in healthcare infrastructure, interdisciplinary training and policy support to optimize the implementation of multidisciplinary approaches. The continued evolution of these models promises to enhance the efficiency and effectiveness of patient care across various healthcare settings.

CASE STUDY

The multidisciplinary approach is a cornerstone of modern medical practice, particularly in complex oncological cases. This case study highlights a successful multidisciplinary collaboration in managing a patient with recurrent brain metastasis from breast cancer, emphasizing the critical role of coordinated medical teamwork (Neagoe, 2022).

Patient Presentation and Initial Diagnosis

A 58-year-old right-handed female patient with a history of stage IIIB breast cancer underwent a radical mastectomy followed by chemotherapy and radiotherapy. The patient also had a history of a left frontoparietal brain metastasis, previously resected. Approximately 4 months after the last intervention, she presented with an epileptic seizure, predominant motor dysphasia and slight right brachial paresis.

Multidisciplinary Assessment

Upon admission, an MDT—including a neurologist, neurosurgeon, radiologist, pathologist, oncologist, anaesthesiologist and radiotherapist—collaborated to evaluate the case. A brain computed tomography (CT) scan and magnetic resonance imaging (MRI) confirmed a recurrence of the left frontoparietal tumour. Given the patient's history, a neurosurgical intervention was deemed necessary.

Neurosurgical Intervention and Postoperative Care

The patient underwent a subtotal resection of the tumour, with a small remnant left due to its adherence to the Sylvian vein vessels. Postoperatively, the patient exhibited mild motor aphasia and right hemiparesis. A comprehensive postoperative rehabilitation plan was implemented, involving neurological assessment, speech therapy and physical rehabilitation.

Role of Each Specialist in the Team

- **Neurologist**: Led the initial neurological assessment and monitored post-surgical recovery, ensuring cognitive and motor functions were preserved.
- **Neurosurgeon**: Performed the tumour resection while balancing the need for maximal tumour removal with the preservation of critical neurological structures.
- **Radiologist**: Provided imaging interpretations that guided surgical decision-making and postoperative monitoring.
- **Pathologist**: Conducted histopathological examinations to confirm tumour recurrence and characterize its molecular profile.
- **Oncologist**: Determined the need for additional systemic therapy post-surgery, adjusting the treatment plan according to the patient's response.
- **Radiotherapist**: Reviewed the feasibility of re-irradiation and collaborated on alternative strategies given prior radiation exposure.
- **Anaesthesiologist**: Ensured optimal perioperative management, minimizing risks associated with brain surgery in a patient with prior oncological treatments.

Outcomes and Follow-Up

The patient showed gradual improvement in motor function and speech postoperatively. Regular follow-up appointments with imaging studies were scheduled to monitor disease progression. Due to prior radiotherapy, the team opted for close observation and systemic therapy rather than additional radiation.

Key Takeaways and Lessons Learned

This case underscores the value of a well-coordinated multidisciplinary approach in managing complex oncological cases. The seamless integration of expertise from multiple specialties facilitated timely decision-making, optimized surgical outcomes and enhanced patient recovery. Effective multidisciplinary collaboration remains the gold standard in ensuring optimal patient care, particularly in cases where standard radiotherapy is not an option.

This case highlights that the key to successful medical intervention lies in structured teamwork, where each specialist's expertise contributes to the patient's overall wellbeing.

BUILDING A NO-RT NETWORK

Building a non-hierarchical (no radiation therapy [NO-RT]) network involves a structured approach that prioritizes collaboration, decentralized decision-making and adaptability. These networks enable organizations, particularly small- and medium-sized enterprises (SMEs), to operate effectively in dynamic environments. The following steps outline the key elements necessary for establishing a NO-RT network.

Step 1: Establish Clear Objectives

The foundation of a NO-RT network begins with defining clear and collaborative objectives. This includes:

- Identifying the overarching goals of the network to ensure alignment with non-hierarchical principles.
- Recognizing key stakeholders and their roles while ensuring equal participation and decision-making authority.
- Emphasizing adaptability and knowledge-sharing mechanisms that support a dynamic and evolving network (Kankaanpaa et al., 2010).

Clearly defining these objectives helps in creating a common vision that fosters trust and cooperation among network participants.

Step 2: Develop a Methodology

A structured methodology enhances the effectiveness of a NO-RT network. One approach involves:

- Adopting frameworks like the Net-Challenge project, which supports SMEs in forming non-hierarchical networks for complex manufacturing (Kankaanpaa et al., 2010).
- Implementing self-organizing principles, wherein network elements adapt and communicate dynamically (Borschbach et al., 2002).
- Utilizing power distribution analysis techniques, such as Markov chains, to ensure balanced decision-making and prevent dominance by specific entities (Andres & Poler, 2014).

By employing these methodological frameworks, NO-RT networks can function more efficiently, leveraging decentralized decision-making for optimal collaboration.

Step 3: Foster Communication and Trust

A key challenge in non-hierarchical networks is maintaining effective communication and trust among participants. This can be achieved by:

- Establishing open and decentralized communication platforms that enable seamless information sharing.
- Encouraging participatory decision-making to enhance network resilience and adaptability.
- Drawing inspiration from decentralized communication methods, such as those used in non-hierarchical personal communication networks, to improve trust and transparency (Bild, 2014).

Trust-building mechanisms, including transparent data-sharing policies and collaborative decision-making processes, strengthen network cohesion and long-term sustainability.

Step 4: Pilot Collaborative Projects

Before scaling the network, it is essential to test its functionality through pilot projects. These projects allow members to:

- Evaluate collaboration dynamics and refine processes based on real-world challenges.
- Apply lessons from successful case studies, such as the LATAM Colorectal Surgery Consortium, which demonstrated the effectiveness of cross-border collaboration in healthcare research (Avellaneda & Smart, 2023).
- Identify potential barriers to cooperation, including cultural differences and infrastructural limitations.

Pilot initiatives serve as valuable learning experiences, providing insights into the network's strengths and areas for improvement.

Step 5: Implement a Roadmap for Growth

For a NO-RT network to achieve long-term sustainability, a structured roadmap should be developed. This includes:

- Following NHNmap, a model designed to transition organizations towards collaborative relationships by outlining development phases and addressing key barriers (Andres & Poler, 2014).
- Establishing fair profit- and cost-sharing models that ensure equitable distribution of resources among participants (Andres & Poler, 2014).
- Incorporating continuous feedback mechanisms to enable iterative improvements in network performance and stakeholder satisfaction (Shamsuzzoha et al., 2012).

A well-defined roadj145map provides a strategic framework for network expansion while maintaining adherence to non-hierarchical principles.

GLOBAL PERSPECTIVES ON NO-RT COLLABORATION

International collaboration has emerged as a transformative model in surgical care, enabling experts from diverse regions to overcome localized resource limitations and regulatory challenges. One notable example is the LATAM Colorectal Surgery Consortium, which brings together specialists from several Latin American countries under a non-hierarchical, decentralized framework. This approach encourages open communication, shared decision-making and the pooling of resources, ultimately enhancing patient outcomes (Kumar et al., 2024).

LATAM Colorectal Surgery Consortium

The LATAM Colorectal Surgery Consortium exemplifies how a collaborative initiative can bridge geographic and systemic divides. By uniting experts from various Latin American nations, the consortium fosters an environment where knowledge and best practices are freely exchanged. This non-hierarchical structure minimizes bureaucratic delays and empowers surgeons to develop innovative, region-specific treatment protocols. The initiative's success lies in its commitment to transparency and inclusivity, which enhances surgical care quality while adapting to the unique challenges of each country (Roberti et al., 2024).

Additional International Initiatives

In addition to the LATAM model, other international collaborations are emerging to further decentralize decision-making in healthcare. A hypothetical initiative, the International Collaborative Oncology Network, illustrates how decentralized strategies can extend beyond regional boundaries. This network would integrate oncology specialists from various continents, creating a platform for cross-cultural knowledge exchange and collective problem-solving. By leveraging the expertise of a globally diverse team, such networks can address complex clinical scenarios and develop adaptable care protocols that are sensitive to local needs (Crippa et al., 2024).

Key Benefits of International Collaboration

International collaborative initiatives bring several critical benefits to surgical care. First, they enhance team-based decision-making by incorporating diverse clinical perspectives, which results in more comprehensive and innovative treatment strategies (Kumar et al., 2024). The sharing of expertise and resources across borders helps mitigate regional disparities, allowing institutions to overcome limitations related to equipment, personnel and funding. Additionally, the cross-cultural exchange inherent in these collaborations fosters a more adaptable and robust approach to patient care, as protocols are continuously refined based on collective insights and varied experiences.

Challenges and Considerations

While the benefits are significant, international collaborations also face challenges. Differing regulatory environments and cultural variations can impede the standardization of treatment protocols and complicate communication among diverse teams. To address these issues, initiatives like the LATAM Consortium and similar networks employ a NO-RT approach that emphasizes decentralized, transparent decision-making. This approach not only facilitates flexible communication strategies but also helps navigate regulatory complexities and cultural differences, ensuring that collaborative efforts remain effective and sustainable (Calkins et al., 2024; Lorona et al., 2024).

By uniting experts through decentralized frameworks, international collaborations such as the LATAM Colorectal Surgery Consortium and emerging networks like the International Collaborative Oncology Network provide a promising model for overcoming regional limitations and advancing global patient care.

ETHICAL DILEMMA: ELDERLY PATIENT DECLINES RADIATION THERAPY

Scenario Overview

An 80-year-old patient, Mr. H, who has been diagnosed with early-stage non-small cell lung cancer (NSCLC), is advised by the oncology team to undergo adjuvant RT following a lobectomy. Despite robust clinical evidence supporting improved local control with RT, Mr. H declines further treatment due to concerns about potential side effects (e.g., fatigue, skin reactions) and a strong personal preference for maintaining his current quality of life. He expresses worries about the impact of RT on his independence and daily functioning.

Ethical Considerations

This scenario raises several ethical challenges for the MDT.

Autonomy vs. Beneficence

While clinicians are obligated to recommend treatments that maximize survival and local control (beneficence), they must also respect the patient's right to refuse treatment (autonomy). The tension here lies in ensuring that Mr. H's decision is truly informed and not unduly influenced by fears or misunderstandings about the therapy.

Informed Consent and Shared Decision-Making

A comprehensive informed consent process is critical. The MDT, which includes thoracic surgeons, medical oncologists, radiation oncologists and palliative care specialists, must provide clear, balanced information about the benefits of adjuvant RT, the associated risks and alternative strategies. Shared decision-making tools (e.g., decision aids or patient education materials) can help ensure that Mr. H is making a choice aligned with his values and that all options are carefully considered.

Quality-of-Life Considerations

In elderly patients, the potential longevity benefit of RT may be offset by its impact on quality of life. The MDT must weigh survival gains against the possibility of additional treatments that could diminish a patient's functional status or result in adverse effects, thus highlighting the significance of patient-centred care.

Multidisciplinary Input and Communication

Regular tumour board meetings and interdisciplinary rounds are essential to integrate various specialties' insights. In Mr. H's case, involving a geriatric specialist and palliative care consultant can provide broader perspectives on managing comorbidities and preserving quality of life, ensuring that the final treatment decision respects both clinical evidence and patient values.

HYPOTHETICAL MALPRACTICE/LEGAL CASE EXAMPLE FROM RT OMISSION

Case Background

In a hypothetical legal case from a mid-sized community hospital, an elderly woman, Mrs. S (aged 78), with early-stage breast cancer initially underwent lumpectomy and was subsequently advised to receive adjuvant RT based on guidelines from studies like CALGB 9343. However, due to inadequate counselling and incomplete documentation, Mrs. S misunderstood the risks and benefits. She independently declined RT without fully grasping the implications regarding local recurrence risks.

Allegations and Ethical/Litigation Issues—Inadequate Informed Consent

The core of the malpractice claim revolved around the allegation that the MDT failed to effectively communicate all relevant information. The legal claim argued that Mrs. S was not provided with comprehensive details—including statistical risks of recurrence without RT and potential benefits—thus undermining her capacity to make an informed decision.

Failure to Document Discussions

In this case, the lack of detailed documentation in the EHR regarding the risks and benefits discussed was a critical factor. Without thorough documentation, it became challenging for the legal defence to prove that informed consent was achieved.

Multidisciplinary Breakdown

The legal claim also cited a breakdown in communication among the team members. Radiologists, pathologists and oncologists held separate discussions with the patient, which were not synthesized into a unified message. This fragmentation contributed to confusion, ultimately culminating in the patient's decision to decline RT.

Legal and Lessons Learned Outcome

The case was settled out of court. The settlement emphasized the hospital's commitment to improving the documentation and delivery of informed consent. It also led to policy changes ensuring that all multidisciplinary decisions and patient interactions are recorded centrally.

Key Lessons for the MDT

Enhanced Communication

Implementation of standardized reporting procedures and coordinated multidisciplinary meetings could mitigate similar issues. Regular tumour board meetings and integrated EHR systems are essential for ensuring that the patient receives a consistent message from all care team members (Mangada et al., 2023).

Robust Informed Consent Process

Incorporating decision aids and involving multiple specialists (including a patient advocate or geriatric specialist) can help ensure that the patient understands the full spectrum of risks and benefits.

Documentation and Follow-Up

Rigorous documentation of patient discussions, especially in instances where treatment deviation (such as RT omission) occurs, is key to demonstrating that the patient was thoroughly informed, a critical factor in malpractice litigation.

Broader Implications

Such a case underscores the importance of a truly multidisciplinary approach that not only integrates clinical expertise but also prioritizes patient education and documentation. It serves as a reminder that, even in cases where patients decline recommended treatments, the responsibility remains with the healthcare team to ensure clarity and unity in their messaging and exhaustive documentation to protect both the patient's interests and the clinician's practice.

CONCLUSION

Creating a NO-RT network requires a structured approach that emphasizes clear objectives, methodological rigor, open communication and sustainable collaboration. While these steps provide a robust framework, challenges such as competitive tensions and cultural differences may arise. Addressing these barriers through continuous dialogue and adaptive strategies is crucial for ensuring the success of a NO-RT network.

REFERENCES

Alsubaie, S. S., Bukhamseen, Z. F. A., Alyami, F. S. A., Alotaibi, M. F., Alkahtani, F. A., Alkhamsan, M. S., Alaseel, A. J., Albahri, M. A. S., Bahrani, J. I. A. A., & Khamees, Z. H. A. (2024). Multidisciplinary approaches in general medical practice: Enhancing collaboration for better patient care. *Journal of Ecohumanism*, *3*(7). https://doi.org/10.62754/joe.v3i7.4665

Amat, N., Jeffery, L., Ann, C. C., Sien, Y. W., Fadzli, A. N., Kuppusamy, S., Saad, M., & Aik, O. T. (2024). The impact of uro-oncology multidisciplinary team meeting (MDTM) on clinical decision-making and adherence to MDTM recommendation: Experience from a tertiary referral centre in Malaysia. *African Journal of Urology*, *30*(1), 12. https://doi.org/10.1186/s12301-024-00415-4

Andrés, B., & Poler, R. (2014). A methodology to share profits and costs in non- hierarchical networks. In J. C. Prado-Prado & J. García-Arca (Eds.), *Annals of Industrial Engineering 2012* (pp. 341–349). Springer London. https://doi.org/10.1007/978-1-4471-5349-8_40

Ardi, B. M., Nursalam, N., & Rosyid, A. N. (2023). Integrated care plan in the hospital setting: A scoping review. *Medical Technology and Public Health Journal*, *7*(2), 171–181. https://doi.org/10.33086/mtphj.v7i2.4733

Avellaneda, N., & Smart, N. J. (2023). Creating a collaborative network in a low/middle income country region. A practical (and motivational) guide to getting started. *Colorectal Disease*, *25*(1), 6–8. https://doi.org/10.1111/codi.16479

Balaratnam, M. S., Rugg-Gunn, F. J., Okin, R., Powell, F., Prior, S., Petrochilos, P., Shivji, D., Haider, S., Alim-Marvasti, A., Chandratheva, A., Simister, R., Lane, C., Macarimban, R., Kaski, D., Athwal, B., Liu, R., Yates, T., Rajakulendran, S., Christofi, G., … Turner, C. (2024). An integrated approach to neuroscience care: An innovative model to support the new integrated care system. *Clinical Medicine*, *24*(6), 100234. https://doi.org/10.1016/j.clinme.2024.100234

Bild, D. R. (2014). *Non-hierarchical networks for censorship-resistant personal communication.* [Thesis]. http://deepblue.lib.umich.edu/handle/2027.42/107314

Borschbach, M., Jansen, R., Freisleben, B., & Lippe, W. (2002). *Non-hierarchical self-organizing network has elements forming cells and each producing logical record with connection data and passing to immediately adjacent neighbors* (Germany Patent No. DE10064874A1). https://patents.google.com/patent/DE10064874A1/en

Calkins, C. M., Rentea, R. M., Smith, C. A., Durham, M. M., & Rideout, D. A. (2024). The pediatric colorectal and pelvic learning consortium. *Journal of Pediatric Surgery*, *59*(8), 1631–1632. https://doi.org/10.1016/j.jpedsurg.2024.04.008

Cenedesi, R. T. F., Moura-Ferreira, M. C. D., Almeida, E. P. F. D., & Júnior, M. A. C. (2024). Effective communication in health: Strategies for effective work development. *IOSR Journal of Humanities and Social Science*, *29*(9), 47–53. https://doi.org/10.9790/0837-2909084753

Chatterjee, D. R., & Mishra, D. V. (2024). Collaborative strategies: Pediatricians and oncologists unite for pediatric cancer management. In T. Elango, Z. A. Bhat, D. S. K. Kar, H. Mulla, S. Chanda, N. Mishra, S. Das, A. Priyadarshini, S. Mahapatra, R. Kumar, A. Garg, P. Shakya, S. Mukherjee, G. Jadhav, D. S. P. Kulkarni, & M. Farooque (Eds.), *Futuristic Trends in Medical Sciences Volume 3 Book 1* (1st ed., pp. 132–134). Iterative International Publisher, Selfypage Developers Pvt Ltd. https://doi.org/10.58532/V3BFMS1P3CH10

Costa, D. K., & Manojlovich, M. (2024). Navigating communication conflicts among the healthcare team. In K. Lalwani, I. Todd Cohen, E. Y. Choi, B. Robins & J. Kirsch (Eds.), *Professional, Ethical, Legal, and Educational Lessons in Medicine* (1st ed., pp. 3–9). Oxford University Press, New York. https://doi.org/10.1093/med/9780197655979.003.0001

Crippa, J., Magistro, C., Montroni, I., Borroni, G., Ziccarelli, A., Spinelli, A., & Mari, G. M. (2024). Charting connections: A systematic review of colorectal surgery research networks. *European Journal of Surgical Oncology*, *50*(6), 108322. https://doi.org/10.1016/j.ejso.2024.108322

Daniel, K. E., Blackstone, S. R., Tan, J. S., Merkel, R. L., Hauck, F. R., & Allen, C. W. (2023). Integrated model of primary and mental healthcare for the refugee population served by an academic medical centre. *Family Medicine and Community Health*, *11*(2), e002038. https://doi.org/10.1136/fmch-2022-002038

DeFilipp, Z., Ciurea, S. O., Cutler, C., Robin, M., & the ASTCT Committee on Practice Guidelines. (2023). Hematopoietic cell transplantation in the management of myelodysplastic syndrome: An evidence-based review from the ASTCT Committee on practice guidelines. *Transplantation and Cellular Therapy*, *29*(2), S2666–6367. https://doi.org/10.1016/j.jtct.2022.11.014

Dobrozsi, S., Trowbridge, A., Mack, J. W., & Rosenberg, A. R. (2019). Effective communication for newly diagnosed pediatric patients with cancer: Considerations for the patients, family members, providers, and multidisciplinary team. *American Society of Clinical Oncology Educational Book*, *39*, 573–581. https://doi.org/10.1200/EDBK_238181

Eaton, V., Zambrano, A., Sanabria, V., Lopez, R., Kyei, I., Mra, R., Sarchet, V., Kremzier, M., Borras, J., Aung, T. K., Morton Doherty, R., Henshall, S., & Camacho, R. (2022). Innovative methodology for strengthening a multidisciplinary team approach in cities in low- and middle-income countries. *JCO Global Oncology*, *8*, e2200149. https://doi.org/10.1200/GO.22.00149

Elsaadi, N. J., & Jahany, M. O. A. (2023). An investigative analysis of the role of multidisciplinary teams in cancer management: Assessing advantages and obstacles. *Scientific Journal of University of Benghazi, 36*(1). https://doi.org/10.37376/sjuob.v36i1.3940

Horgan, D., Van Den Bulcke, M., Malats, N., De Maria, R., Dube, F., Singh, J., Hofman, P., Omar, M. I., Malapelle, U., Hills, T., Pepe, F., & Subbiah, V. (2024). Understanding the landscape of cancer care in Europe: Evaluating clinical and comprehensive cancer centers. *Healthcare, 12*(23), 2338. https://doi.org/10.3390/healthcare12232338

Kankaanpaa, T., Shamsuzzoha, A., Carneiro, L., Almeida, R., Helo, P., Fornasiero, R., Ferreira, P. S., & Chiodi, A. (2010). Methodology for non-hierarchical collaboration networks for complex products manufacturing. *2010 IEEE International Technology Management Conference (ICE)*, 1–10. https://doi.org/10.1109/ICE.2010.7477018

King, H. B., Battles, J., Baker, D. P., Alonso, A., Salas, E., Webster, J., Toomey, L., & Salisbury, M. (2008). Teamstepps™: Team strategies and tools to enhance performance and patient safety. In K. Henriksen, J. B. Battles, M. A. Keyes & M. L. Grady (Eds.), *Advances in Patient Safety: New Directions and Alternative Approaches (Vol. 3: Performance and Tools)*. Agency for Healthcare Research and Quality (US). http://www.ncbi.nlm.nih.gov/books/NBK43686/

Kumar, N., Hyman, G. Y., Gerk, A., Wurdeman, T., Uribe-Leitz, T., Corlew, S., Park, K. B., Meara, J. G., Riviello, R., Makasa, E. M., Kolker, J., Manrique, J., Ayala, R. E., Ibbotson, G. C., Mejia, A., Falcão, L. F., Fuentes, M. J. G., Montalvo-Samaniego, M., Baki, I. A., … Vega, A. B. (2024). Scalable policy adoption and sustainable implementation of surgical care in the Americas. *Revista Panamericana de Salud Pública, 48*, 1. https://doi.org/10.26633/RPSP.2024.132

Lobo, A. F. R., & daPalma, T. M. R. (2024). The importance of multidisciplinary teams in healthcare: Critical analysis and reflection. *Revista Ibero-Americana de Humanidades, Ciências e Educação, 10*(11), 3853–3859. https://doi.org/10.51891/rease.v10i11.16749

Lorona, M. E., Pérez, G., Martínez, R., Gómez, L., & Alvarez, J. (2024). Building collaborative oncology networks: Overcoming regional disparities through decentralized approaches. *Global Oncology Journal, 10*(2), 145–153.

Mangada, K. L., Moffet, J., Nishitani, M., Albuquerque, S., & Duncan, C. N. (2023). Interprofessional team-based care of the hematopoietic cell transplantation patient with hepatic veno-occlusive disease/sinusoidal obstruction syndrome. *Journal of Pediatric Hematology/Oncology, 45*(1), 12–17. https://doi.org/10.1097/MPH.0000000000002594

Mangone, L., Zizzo, M., Nardecchia, M., Marinelli, F., Bisceglia, I., Braghiroli, M. B., Banzi, M. C., Damato, A., Cerullo, L., Pellegri, C., Morabito, F., Neri, A., Fabozzi, M., Pinto, C., & Giorgi Rossi, P. (2024). Impact of multidisciplinary team management on survival and recurrence in stage i–iii colorectal cancer: A population-based study in Northern Italy. *Biology, 13*(11), 928. https://doi.org/10.3390/biology13110928

Neagoe, M.-A. (2022). Multidisciplinary collaboration the gold standard of medical practice. *International Journal of Advanced Research, 10*(03), 1092–1094. https://doi.org/10.21474/IJAR01/14494

Parker, P. A., Staley, J., Rosa, W. E., Weiner, R., & Banerjee, S. C. (2024). Development of a communication skills training to enhance effective team communication in oncology. *Journal of Continuing Education in the Health Professions, 44*(1), 71–74. https://doi.org/10.1097/CEH.0000000000000503

Roberti, J., Rodríguez, V., Seijo, M., Rodríguez, A. P., Guglielmino, M., Jorro-Barón, F., Baigorria, M. D. L. A., Villa, S., Cornistein, W., Ocampo, C. V., Clara, L., Colque, M., Staneloni, M. I., Piccinini, P., Pidal, P., Bagnulo, H., Albornoz, H., Vivas, C., Pike, P., & García-Elorrio, E. (2024). Modified Delphi RAND/UCLA consensus on recommendations for preventing surgical site infections in colorectal surgery: A multimodal approach in Latin America. *Infectious Diseases in Clinical Practice, 32*(4). https://doi.org/10.1097/IPC.0000000000001373

Schroeder, E., Lynch, K., & Turgeon, A. (2017). Strategies for effective collaboration among multidisciplinary teams: Integration of an ABA professional [Reports]. Student Research and Creative Works. University of Puget Sound. https://jstor.org/stable/community.36514200

Shamsuzzoha, A. H. M., Kankaanpää, T., Carneiro, L., & Almeida, R. (2012). Methodological support to establish a collaborative non-hierarchical business network for complex product manufacturing. *International Journal of Networking and Virtual Organisations*, *11*(3/4), 363. https://doi.org/10.1504/IJNVO.2012.048926

Sugiyama, A., Utsunomiya, K., Okumiya, H., Fujimoto, K., Shimomura, Y., Sanuki, M., Kume, K., Yano, T., Kagawa, R., & Bando, H. (2024). Toward a patient-centered care supporting system: Integration of multidisciplinary health records in breast cancer care. In J. Mantas, A. Hasman, G. Demiris, K. Saranto, M. Marschollek, T. N. Arvanitis, I. Ognjanović, A. Benis, P. Gallos, E. Zoulias, & E. Andrikopoulou (Eds.), *Studies in Health Technology and Informatics*. IOS Press. https://doi.org/10.3233/SHTI240756

Suh, M., & Cheon, G. J. (2024). Multidisciplinary team approach in prostate-specific membrane antigen theranostics for prostate cancer: A narrative review. *Journal of Urologic Oncology*, *22*(1), 11–20. https://doi.org/10.22465/juo.244600200010

Tullis, J. A. (2022). Tumor talk: A descriptive study of communication about tumor board meetings. *Qualitative Research in Medicine and Healthcare*, *6*(2). https://doi.org/10.4081/qrmh.2022.10717

CHAPTER 10

Concluding Remarks

Using NO-RT in a Holistic Cancer Treatment Approach

Rahul Jain, Rahul Sapate and Vishal Gulecha

KEY CONCEPTS

As we conclude this exploration of the no radiation therapy (NO-RT) approach, it becomes evident that a shift is underway in how we think about cancer treatment. Across this book, we've examined how advancements in diagnostics, systemic therapies and molecular biology are challenging the once-default reliance on radiation therapy. This chapter brings together the key concepts and guiding principles that have emerged throughout, offering a consolidated understanding of how oncology is evolving in real time.

Throughout this book, several unifying principles have emerged. First, the importance of individualized care—driven by patient biology, preferences and prognosis—has been central to the NO-RT philosophy. The clinical evidence supports that RT is not always necessary, especially when modern systemic therapies and surgical advances offer equivalent or better outcomes with fewer side effects.

Second, tumour biology and molecular profiling now guide treatment planning more than ever before. Technologies like genetic assays and biomarker analysis allow clinicians to better identify patients who may safely avoid radiation.

Third, the book emphasized a patient-centred approach that values quality of life alongside survival outcomes. The growing body of data from global trials and real-world evidence confirms that reducing or eliminating radiation, when appropriate, can preserve function, dignity and wellbeing.

Finally, the NO-RT strategy calls for a thoughtful recalibration of oncology protocols. It does not advocate for abandoning radiation entirely, but rather for its selective and justified use based on evolving science. This approach requires multidisciplinary collaboration, continuous education and openness to changing long-standing norms.

DOI: 10.1201/9781003529071-10

NO-RT's ROLE IN HOLISTIC CANCER CARE

- *Reduced Morbidity*: Radiation therapy, while highly effective, often causes significant side effects, including fatigue, nausea, skin reactions and organ damage. These side effects can dramatically affect a patient's quality of life, affecting their ability to work, engage in social activities and maintain overall wellbeing. NO-RT, by minimizing or eliminating radiation, directly addresses this concern, leading to improved physical functioning and reduced symptom burden. This allows patients to maintain a better quality of life during and after treatment.
- *Enhanced Quality of Life*: The focus on quality of life is paramount in holistic cancer care, and NO-RT directly contributes to this goal. By reducing treatment-related toxicity, NO-RT allows patients to experience fewer disruptions to their daily lives, participate more fully in their social networks and maintain a greater sense of normalcy. This is particularly crucial in managing long-term effects and improving overall wellbeing.
- *Personalized Treatment Plans*: Holistic care demands personalized treatment plans tailored to individual patient needs. NO-RT supports this by allowing clinicians to consider not only the tumour characteristics but also the patient's overall health, age, preferences and potential for complications. This personalized approach ensures the chosen treatment aligns with the patient's unique circumstances and goals, leading to improved patient satisfaction and adherence. The decision to forgo radiation is not taken lightly, but rather made through rigorous evaluation and shared decision-making, ensuring autonomy.
- *Improved Patient–Clinician Communication*: A holistic approach necessitates open and honest communication between clinicians and patients. NO-RT fosters this by encouraging discussions about the risks and benefits of radiation versus other treatment modalities. This collaborative decision-making process empowers patients to be active participants in their care, leading to greater trust and a stronger therapeutic alliance. Transparency and informed consent are key to successful integration.
- *Multidisciplinary Care*: Holistic cancer care typically involves a multidisciplinary team (MDT) that includes oncologists, surgeons, nurses, social workers, psychologists and other specialists. NO-RT naturally fits within this framework, requiring collaboration among team members to assess patient suitability, plan alternative therapies and manage potential complications. The MDT ensures comprehensive care, addressing the patient's multifaceted needs.

FUTURE OUTLOOK FOR NO-RT IN ONCOLOGY

- *Technological Advancements*: Continued improvements in surgical techniques (minimally invasive procedures, robotic surgery); targeted therapies (gene therapy, immunotherapy); and imaging technologies (improved diagnostic capabilities, real-time monitoring) will further expand the applicability of NO-RT. More precise and effective non-radiation alternatives will emerge, reducing the need for radiation in more cases.
- *Biomarker Discovery*: Advances in genomic sequencing and proteomics will enable the identification of more precise biomarkers that predict treatment response and identify

patients who are likely to benefit from NO-RT. This will allow for more accurate patient selection and reduce the risk of treatment failure due to inadequate response.

- *Artificial Intelligence (AI)*: AI-driven decision support systems will play an increasingly important role in guiding treatment decisions and optimizing NO-RT strategies. AI can analyse complex datasets to predict treatment outcomes and personalize treatment plans, ensuring appropriate candidate selection and maximizing treatment efficacy.
- *Clinical Trials and Research*: Further robust clinical trials are needed to validate the effectiveness of NO-RT in various cancer types and patient populations. These studies should focus not only on survival rates but also on quality of life, long-term complications and cost-effectiveness. This will help establish evidence-based guidelines and protocols for the implementation of NO-RT in clinical practice.

FUTURE DIRECTIONS IN CLINICAL TRIALS AND RESEARCH

As NO-RT evolves from a promising concept to a standard component of holistic cancer care, robust clinical trials and innovative research designs are essential to confirm its efficacy, optimize patient selection and integrate emerging technologies. Rigorous clinical studies not only validate the benefits of NO-RT but also offer insights into long-term quality of life, cost-effectiveness and overall treatment outcomes. Advancing our understanding through these trials will support the evolution of NO-RT into a widely accepted, patient-centred approach to cancer management.

MULTICENTER AND RANDOMIZED CONTROLLED TRIALS

Conducting large-scale, multi-institutional randomized controlled trials is critical for comparing NO-RT strategies with traditional RT. These studies, spanning diverse populations and treatment settings, will establish the safety, efficacy and generalizability of NO-RT protocols, thereby building a robust evidence base to guide clinical practice.

ADAPTIVE TRIAL DESIGNS

Incorporating adaptive trial designs enables real-time modifications based on emerging data. By allowing interim analyses and flexible adjustments to study protocols, adaptive trials can quickly identify optimal treatment regimens. This innovative approach reduces delays in translating research findings into effective patient care, ensuring that the most promising strategies are implemented promptly.

BIOMARKER-DRIVEN PATIENT SELECTION

Integrating molecular profiling and genetic biomarkers into clinical trial protocols is essential for refining patient selection. A biomarker-driven strategy enhances patient stratification by identifying individuals most likely to benefit from NO-RT. This targeted methodology minimizes the risk of adverse outcomes and improves the overall efficiency of clinical trials by ensuring appropriate candidate enrolment.

INTEGRATION OF AI AND MACHINE LEARNING

Leveraging AI and machine learning in clinical trial analytics offers a transformative approach to analysing complex datasets. These advanced tools can predict treatment responses, uncover hidden patterns and facilitate the customization of care plans. Their integration into research protocols will accelerate the discovery of innovative therapeutic strategies and support personalized treatment approaches.

LONG-TERM OUTCOMES AND QUALITY-OF-LIFE METRICS

Future studies should expand their focus beyond traditional survival endpoints by incorporating long-term outcomes and quality-of-life measures. Including patient-reported outcomes, cost analyses and assessments of chronic morbidity will provide a comprehensive evaluation of NO-RT's impact on patient wellbeing.

In summary, embracing these advanced clinical trial methodologies is paramount for validating NO-RT's benefits and fostering its evolution into a cornerstone of personalized cancer care. Collaboration among researchers, clinicians and industry stakeholders will be key to driving these initiatives forward. Moving forward, it is imperative that the oncology community continues to innovate in trial design and collaborate across disciplines to integrate these advancements seamlessly into clinical practice. By prioritizing multicentre trials and embracing adaptive, data-driven methodologies, researchers will not only accelerate the pace of discovery but also ensure that treatment regimens are finely tuned to individual patient needs. This forward-thinking approach promises to transform cancer care by delivering effective therapies aligned with holistic patient goals.

THE FUTURE OF NO-RT IN ONCOLOGY

The future of NO-RT in oncology holds significant promise as a cornerstone of personalized cancer care. As clinicians and researchers continue to evaluate the efficacy of de-escalation protocols, several critical research questions and potential policy changes emerge that will shape treatment paradigms over the coming decade.

KEY RESEARCH QUESTIONS

To advance the field, a number of research questions need to be addressed through rigorous clinical trials and observational studies.

Long-Term Survival Outcomes

A primary research question is, "What are the long-term survival outcomes of NO-RT in human papillomavirus (HPV)-positive head and neck cancer?" This inquiry is crucial, as early data suggest that immunotherapy and targeted systemic treatments might offer survival benefits comparable to traditional RT, while also reducing long-term toxicities.

Quality of Life and Functional Outcomes

Future studies should examine how NO-RT affects patients' quality of life over extended periods. For example, assessing cognitive function in young brain tumour patients and functional status in elderly patients will help determine whether avoiding RT significantly improves daily living and overall wellbeing.

Biomarker-Driven Patient Selection

Investigations into the role of biomarkers, such as PD-L1 expression and genomic signatures, are needed to refine patient selection. A specific question is, "Can multi-omics profiling reliably predict which patients can safely forgo RT without compromising local control?" These studies will further solidify the use of precision medicine in de-escalation strategies.

Cost-Effectiveness and Healthcare Resource Allocation

Evaluating the cost-effectiveness of NO-RT protocols versus traditional RT remains an open question. Research should explore whether the reduced treatment burden and lower long-term toxicity translate into significant healthcare savings and improved resource allocation.

POTENTIAL POLICY CHANGES

Based on emerging evidence from ongoing trials and real-world data, several policy shifts are anticipated in the near future.

National Guidelines and Standard of Care

By 2030, it is anticipated that national guidelines may evolve to include NO-RT as a recommended option for early-stage cancers. This change would reflect robust evidence from multicentre randomized controlled trials that demonstrate comparable survival outcomes with reduced toxicity in selected patient populations.

Incorporation of Biomarker Testing

As genomic and molecular profiling becomes increasingly integral to treatment planning, policymakers may mandate routine biomarker testing for cancers where NO-RT is a viable option. Such policies would ensure that patients receive personalized treatment recommendations, thereby reducing unnecessary radiation exposure.

Regulatory Acceptance of Adaptive Trial Designs

Regulatory bodies may begin to accept adaptive trial designs that integrate real-time data and multi-omics insights to refine treatment protocols. This policy shift would facilitate more rapid translation of research findings into clinical practice and support the continuous evolution of NO-RT strategies.

Reimbursement and Coverage Adjustments

In tandem with clinical guideline updates, insurance providers and healthcare systems might adjust reimbursement models to incentivize personalized, evidence-based treatments that prioritize patient quality of life. These adjustments could include higher reimbursement rates for genomic testing and AI-driven treatment planning that support NO-RT approaches.

FUTURE DIRECTIONS

Advancements in AI and adaptive radiotherapy are set to further optimize the implementation of NO-RT. AI-driven predictive models that analyse complex datasets encompassing clinical, imaging and molecular data are already enhancing patient selection and treatment planning. This technology promises to refine fractionation schemes and predict treatment outcomes, thereby reducing unnecessary RT exposure. Furthermore, dynamic imaging and real-time adaptive techniques will allow clinicians to adjust treatment protocols based on tumour behaviour, further individualizing care and minimizing toxicity.

In summary, the future of NO-RT in oncology is poised for significant advancement through targeted research and evolving policy. Addressing critical questions about long-term outcomes, quality of life, biomarker efficacy and cost-effectiveness will be essential for integrating NO-RT into standard care practices. As evidence accumulates, policy changes, including updated national guidelines, mandatory biomarker testing, adaptive trial designs and revised reimbursement models, will help ensure that NO-RT becomes a safe, effective and patient-centred approach in the holistic management of cancer. These advancements promise to transform cancer care by reducing treatment burdens, preserving patient quality of life and delivering personalized therapeutic strategies that align with the unique needs of each patient.

UNANSWERED RESEARCH QUESTIONS

Long-Term Survival Outcomes

What are the extended survival benefits of NO-RT protocols compared to conventional RT, particularly across diverse cancer types and patient demographics?

Quality of Life and Functional Metrics

How does the omission of RT affect long-term quality of life, cognitive function and overall physical performance, especially in vulnerable groups such as the elderly and paediatric patients?

Biomarker Validation and Patient Selection

Can emerging genomic and proteomic biomarkers (e.g., PD-L1 expression, multi-omics profiles) be reliably used to select patients who will most benefit from NO-RT without compromising local control?

Cost-Effectiveness and Healthcare Impact

Is the NO-RT approach more cost-effective when considering the reduced toxicity, fewer hospitalizations and potential healthcare savings over time compared to conventional RT?

Integration of AI and Adaptive Technologies

How can AI, advanced imaging and adaptive radiotherapy techniques be further developed and integrated to tailor patient-specific NO-RT strategies effectively?

Long-Term Oncologic Safety and Recurrence Risks

What are the patterns of local and distant recurrence in patients managed without RT over a decade or more, and how do these compare with the standard of care?

PREDICTED NO-RT POLICY SHIFTS BY 2030

Revised National Guidelines

National cancer treatment protocols may formally incorporate NO-RT as a recommended option for selected early-stage cancers once long-term efficacy data become robust.

Mandatory Biomarker Testing

Routine genomic and molecular profiling could become standard practice to guide personalized treatment decisions, ensuring that only patients with favourable profiles are offered NO-RT.

Regulatory Acceptance of Adaptive Trial Designs

Regulatory bodies might endorse adaptive, real-time trial designs that integrate multi-omics and AI data to rapidly update and refine NO-RT treatment protocols.

Reimbursement and Coverage Adjustments

Healthcare payers may adjust reimbursement models to incentivize the use of personalized NO-RT strategies—including higher coverage for advanced diagnostic tests and AI-supported decision-making tools.

Enhanced Multidisciplinary Frameworks

Policy shifts are likely to promote more integrated, team-based care models that leverage comprehensive electronic health records (EHRs) and centralized decision support systems to streamline treatment planning and improve overall patient outcomes.

ANALYSIS SUMMARY

After reviewing the current literature and the evolving landscape of cancer treatment supported by recent advances in biomarker discovery, AI-driven personalized medicine and adaptive clinical trial designs synthesize the key areas where further research is needed and predict how policy may evolve over the next decade to better integrate NO-RT into holistic cancer management. These elements echo emerging trends described in recent studies and consensus statements from leading oncology centres, framing a forward-thinking outlook for how personalized, less toxic treatment paradigms might shape clinical practice by 2030.

CALL TO ACTION

The potential benefits of NO-RT for improving patient outcomes and quality of life are substantial. However, its full potential remains untapped. A concerted call to action is required for clinicians and researchers

Clinicians need to embrace a patient-centred approach that prioritizes individualized treatment plans. They also need to actively engage in shared decision-making with patients to determine the most appropriate treatment strategy, considering NO-RT as a viable option when appropriate.

Index

Note: Page references with *italics* refer to figures, **bold** refers to tables.

5- Fluorouracil (5-FU)-based therapies, 11

A

Access to Advanced Health Institute (AAHI), 71
Acidic extracellular environment, 24
Adaptive radiotherapy, 35–36, 41, 156, 157
Adaptive Response Clinical Decision Support (ARCliDS), 89
Adaptive trial designs, 153, 155
ADAPT-RT, 14
Advanced pancreatic adenocarcinoma (APC), 11
African Organization for Research and Training in Cancer (AORTIC), 70
Algorithm development, 96–97
- clinical decision trees, 96–97
- integration of clinical data, 96
- machine learning applications, 96

Alternative modalities, 62–73
- global disparities in access to, 69
- international collaborations, 69–71
- research networks, 69–71

American Society for Radiation Oncology (ASTRO), 77
American Society of Clinical Oncology (ASCO), 13, 71
American Urological Association (AUA), 100
Anaesthesiologist (role), 141
Apoptosis, 63
Area under the curve (AUC), 30, 79
Artificial intelligence (AI), 34, 89, 153
- driven predictive modelling, 34
- driven treatment planning, 36
- integration of, 154
- in patient selection for NO-RT, 34–35
- role in decision-making of NO-RT, 105
- tools, 73

Asian case study, 118
Autonomy *vs.* beneficence, 145
Axillary lymph node dissection (ALND), 54

B

Beneficence, 83–84, 86, 93, 145
Bias
- cognitive, 89, 97
- data, 97
- subjective, 89

Biochemical alterations, 24
Biochemical disease-free survival (bDFS), 120
Biological compatibility concerns, 133
Biomarkers, 20, 22–23, 29–32, 41, **57**, 152
- clinical application examples of, 32–33
- driven patient selection, 153, 155
- genetic, 29–30, 153
- germline genetic, 29–30
- integration of, 22
- machine learning for, 29
- prognostic, 30–32
- role of, 6
- support RT omission, **57**
- testing, 155

Bragg peaks, 64, 67
Breast cancer, 53, 63, 101; *see also* Cancer
- decision-making algorithm, 104
- disputes, 128
- early-stage, 9, 11, 37, 38, 41, 50, 55, 91–92, 104, 121, 131, 146
- luminal A, 32
- management, 136
- nutritional support in, 66
- Oncotype DX in, 33
- risk stratification, 80
- treatment, 66

Breast-conserving surgery, 6
Breast Health Global Initiative (BHGI), 69
Broader implications, 147

C

CALGB 9343 trials, 38, 41, 50, 51, 53, 57
Cancer; *see also* Breast cancer; Rectal cancer
  bladder, 53–54
  colon, 72
  colorectal, 30, 32, 101
  cost-effective treatments, 68
  gastric, 65, 72
  liver, 65
  MSI-H colorectal, 32
  recurrence, 5
Cancer-associated fibroblasts (CAFs), 24, 28
Cancer stem cells (CSCs), *23*
Cao, B., 8
Capacity building, 70, 71
Care
  coordination of, 137–138
  customization of, 99–100
  individualized, 116
  multidisciplinary, 152
  postoperative, 141
Care models
  integrated, 139–140
  multidisciplinary, 139–140
Case studies, 111–122
  Asian, 118
  early-stage breast cancer without radiation, 55
  European, 117–118
  IDEA trial, 57
  neoadjuvant chemotherapy for locally advanced rectal cancer, 55–56
  omission of radiation therapy, 111–113
  omission of radiotherapy, 111–113
  PRIME II trial, 57
  Royal Marsden Hospital, 117–119
  watch-and-wait (W&W) strategy, 113–115
  watch-and-wait strategy in rectal cancer, 56
Cell proliferation, 63
Central nervous system tumours, 73; *see also* Tumours
Chemokines, 24
Chemoradiotherapy (CRT), 81
Chemotherapy, 3, 53–54, 62–63, 65, 91, 111
  in advanced ovarian cancer, 54
  conventional, 72
  cytotoxic effects, 63
  second-line, 11
  systemic, 8
Chromosome alterations, 26
Circulating tumour DNA (ctDNA), 30
Clinical algorithms, 89
Clinical complete response (cCR), 56, 113
Clinical data integration, 96
Clinical decision trees (CDTs), 96–97
Clinical determination, 89–105; *see also* Decision-making
  additional trials, 92
  challenges/considerations, 103
  clinical pathways, 97–99
  comparative analysis, 92
  customization of care, 99–100
  data collection, 101–102
  documentation, 101–102
  ethical considerations in RT de-escalation, 93–94
  evidence-based recommendations, 102
  implications for clinical practice, 97
  legal implications, 94
  malpractice claims, 94
  monitoring/follow-up, 100
  patient-centric approaches, 100–101
  robust, 103
Clinical efficacy, 132
Clinical guidelines, harmonization of, 70–71
Clinical pathways, 15, 97–99
  development, 98
  integrating NO-RT, 97–99, *98*
  integration of, 98
  promote standardization, 98
Cognitive bias, 97; *see also* Bias
Colon cancer, 72; *see also* Cancer
Colorectal cancer, 30, 32, 101; *see also* Cancer
Communication, 143, 146
  digital tools, 139
  enhanced, 147
  importance of, 117
  improved patient–clinician, 152
  skills, 139
  strategies, 138
Complementary and alternative medicine (CAM), 65
Complete clinical response (cCR), 8
Complete metabolic response (CMR), 111
Comprehensive cancer centres, 139
Computed tomography (CT), 100, 141
Confidence intervals (CIs), 51
Controversies, 127
Convolutional neural networks (CNNs), 99
Coordination of care, 137–138
Cost-effectiveness, 155
  cancer treatments, 68
  of NO-RT, 130–131
  of radiofrequency ablation, 68–69

Cost of systems, 131–132
Coverage adjustments, 155–156
Craniospinal irradiation (CSI), 40
Cultural attitudes, impact of, 119–120
Customization of care, 99–100
Cytokines, 24
Cytoreductive surgery (CRS), 54, 77
  decision algorithm, 104–105
  ideal candidates for, 81
Cytotoxic effects, 63

D

DA-EPOCH-R regimen, 111, 119
Danish Breast Cancer Group (DBCG), 85
Data
  analysis, 103
  bias, 97
  collection, 101–103
  gene expression, 29
  integration, 34, 37, 103
Deauville score (DS), 111
Decipher score, 22, 33
Decision-making; *see also* Clinical determination
  challenges, 96
  data-driven, 95
  frameworks, 89–90
  integration into, 95–96
  from major clinical trials, 90
  multidisciplinary, 91
  shared, 94, 145
  TARGIT-A trial impact on, 91–92
De-escalation trials, 92–94
Defective mismatch repair (dMMR), 30, 32
Diagnostic accuracy, 136
Difficulties/disputations, 123–133
  clinical challenges, 123
  complex eligibility criteria, 123
  controversies, 127
  expectation management, 125
  financial constraints, 124
  human resource challenge, 125
  patient management, 125
  patient selection, 123
  practical/infrastructural barriers, 133
  quality assurance (QA), 124
  regulatory and ethical considerations, 124
  workflow adaptation, 124
Digital communication tools, 139; *see also* Communication
Disease-free survival (DFS), 50, 136
DNA synthesis, 63
Documentation, 138, 147
  clinical determination, 101–102
  importance of, 102–103
  precise, 102
  proper, 103
Doe, John, 121
Dose delivery efficiency, 132
Dose painting, 35–36
Dosimetry, 1
Ductal carcinoma in situ (DCIS), 28
Dynamic imaging, 35, 36

E

Early-stage breast cancer, 9, 11, 37, 38, 41, 50, 55, 91–92, 104, 121, 131, 146; *see also* Breast cancer
Early-stage breast cancer without radiation, case study, 55
Economic disparities, 125–126
Economic impact, 131
Effector cells, 26
Electronic health records (EHRs), 99, 137–138
Eligible trials network, *10*
ENCEPHALON trial, 7
Endocrine therapy (ET), 2, 6, 11, 32, 37–39, 53, 58, 85, 127
Energy delivery/source, 133
Enhanced communication, 147; *see also* Communication
Epithelial-to-mesenchymal transition (EMT), 24, 26
European case study, 117–118
European Society for Medical Oncology (ESMO), 13, 71, 117
European Society for Radiotherapy and Oncology (ESTRO), 12–13, 77
Evidence-based practices, 13, 78, 86, 95, 97–98, 113, 115–116, 131
  build confidence, 116
  framework for, 70
Evidence-based recommendations, 102
Expectation management, 125
Extracellular matrix (ECM), 24

F

Family preferences, 114
Financial constraints, 124
Fluorouracil and oxaliplatin (FOLFOX) chemotherapy, 51
Focused ultrasound (FUS), 63, 64, 66, 68
FOLFIRINOX *vs.* Gemcitabine alone, 10

FOLFOX, 55, 56
Follow-up
  duration, 85
  guidelines, 100
  protocols, 101
Frontline immunochemotherapy, 111

G

Gastric cancer, 65, 72; *see also* Cancer
Gemcitabine plus nab-paclitaxel, 10
Gene expression data, 29; *see also* Data
Genetics
  biomarkers, 29–30, 153
  mutations, 4, 6, 8, 20, 22, 42
  profiling, 6, 20, 29–32, 41
  resistance, 52
  screening, 25
  signatures, 30
  variations, 25
Genomic heterogeneity, 26
Genomic stability, 25
Germline genetic biomarkers, 29–30
Global Alliance for Genomics and Health (GA4GH), 70
Global barriers, 126–127
Global Health Innovative Technology Fund (GHIT), 71
Growth factors, 24
Grubb, E.H., 1
Gynaecologic oncology, 128

H

Haemorrhagic cystitis, 29
Harmonization of clinical guidelines, 70–71
Hazard ratios (HRs), 51
Head and neck cancer, 29–30, 37, 50–52, 62, 67, 77, 80, 92, 101–102, 104, 154
Healthcare implications, 130–131
Healthcare infrastructure, 71, 86, 119, 125, 140
Healthcare resource allocation, 155
Hepatocellular carcinoma (HCC), 65
HER2-negative tumours, 2; *see also* Tumours
High-intensity focused ultrasound (HIFU), 64, 66, 67, 70, 71
Histotripsy, 65, 71–72
Holistic care, 72, 100–102, 152
Holzknecht, Guido, 1
Human papillomavirus (HPV), 154
Human resource challenge, 125
Hyperthermic intraperitoneal, 54
Hyperthermic intraperitoneal chemotherapy (HIPEC), 54, 77, 81
Hypothetical malpractice/legal case, 146–147
Hypoxia, 20–21, 24, 26, *27*, 32–34, 41, 62
Hypoxic environment, 24
Hypoxic tumour microenvironment, 32
Hypoxic tumour response, 26, *27*

I

IBM Watson, 34–35, 73
IDEA trial, 51, 57
IELSG37 trial, 112, 116, 121
Imaging technologies, 3, 4, 152
Immune cell interaction, 26, 27
Immune checkpoint inhibitors (ICIs), 22
Immune heterogeneity, 26
Immunocompromised patients, 82, 86
Immunotherapy, 7, 14, 21–23, 30–33, 41, 62–63, 99, 124, 128, 152
Improved patient–clinician communication, 152; *see also* Communication
Individualized care, 116; *see also* Care
Individualized surveillance, 101
Informed consent, 94, 145
Infrastructural barriers, 133
Infrastructure limitations, 125–126
Institutional expertise, 116
Institutional protocols, 114
Integrated care networks, 140
Integrative oncology, 71, 72
Intensity-modulated radiation therapy (IMRT), 28, 132
Interdisciplinary rounds, 138
International Agency for Research on Cancer (IARC), 83
International Atomic Energy Agency (IAEA), 12–13, 70, 78, 127
International Cancer Genome Consortium (ICGC), 69
International Classification of Diseases, Tenth Edition (ICD-10), 79
International clinical trials, 14
International collaboration, 126, 144
  benefits of, 144
  challenges, 144–145
  initiatives, 144
  LATAM Colorectal Surgery Consortium, 144
  NO-RT, 144–145
International Collaborative Oncology Network, 144
International disparities, 131
International initiatives, 144

International Organization for Standardization (ISO), 126
International standards/guidelines suitability, 77–79
Intraoperative radiotherapy (IORT), 91
Ipsilateral breast tumour recurrence (IBTR), 11, 91

L

Laparoscopic surgery, 53; *see also* Surgery
LATAM Colorectal Surgery Consortium, 144
Leukaemia, 1
Liver cancer, 65; *see also* Cancer
Local ablative therapy (LAT), 12
Localized tumours, 52; *see also* Tumours
Locally advanced rectal cancer (LARC), 8
Long-term monitoring, 115
Long-term outcomes, 154
Long-term survival outcomes, 154
Long-term toxicity management expenses, 130
Low- and middle-income countries (LMICs), 13, 69–70, 125–126, 131, 137
Luminal A breast cancer, 32; *see also* Cancer
LUMINA trial, 2, 37, 39, 84, 92
  age restriction, 85
  highly selective cohort, 85
  limitations of, 84–85
  short follow-up duration, 85
Lumpectomy, 53
Lung cancer
  non-surgical approaches in, 39
  PD-L1 expression in, 32
  prognostic biomarkers in, 30–32

M

Machine learning (ML), 95, 154
  applications, 96
  for biomarker discovery, 29
  evolution of, 96
Magnetic resonance imaging (MRI), 100, 113, 141
Mammography, 128
Marincaş, A.M., 104
Matrix metalloproteinases (MMPs), 24
MD Anderson Cancer Center, 139
Memorial Sloan Kettering Cancer Center, 139
Microsatellite instability (MSI), 22
Minimally invasive surgery (MIS), 52–53
Molecular profiling, 3–4, 6, 12–13, 22, 38, 52, 99, 105, 129, 151, 153, 155, 157
Monitoring/follow-up, 100
MR-guided radiotherapy (MRgRT), 123, 124–125, 129–130
MSI-H colorectal cancer, 32; *see also* Cancer
Multicriteria optimization, 35–36
Multidisciplinary assessment, 141
Multidisciplinary breakdown, 146
Multidisciplinary care, 152
Multidisciplinary clinics, 139
Multidisciplinary collaboration, 116
Multidisciplinary cooperation, 136–147
  case study, 140–142
  communication strategies, 138
  ethical dilemma, 145–146
  global perspectives on NO-RT collaboration, 144–145
  hypothetical malpractice/legal case, 146–147
  integrated care models, 139–140
  NO-RT network, 142–143
  regular tumour board meetings, 138–139
  team-based approach, 136–138
Multidisciplinary decision-making, 91
Multidisciplinary input, 146
Multidisciplinary team (MDT), 82–83, 86, 136–137, 147, 152
Multidisciplinary team meetings (MDTMs), 136
Multidisciplinary tumour boards (MTBs), 91
Multimodal imaging, 35
Myeloid cells, 24, 27
Myeloid-derived suppressor cells (MDSCs), 27
Myxoid liposarcomas, 12

N

Nanogram, 76–77, 80
National Comprehensive Cancer Network (NCCN), 70, 78
National Oncology Societies, 13
NATURAL trial, 85
Neoadjuvant chemotherapy for locally advanced rectal cancer, case study, 55–56
Neoadjuvant therapy (NAT), 8, 81
Neurocognitive concerns, 40
Neurologic, oncologic, mechanical instability and systemic disease (NOMS), 89
Neurologist (role), 141
Neurosurgeon (role), 141
Neurosurgical intervention, 141
New England Journal of Medicine, 121
Nomogram, 77, 80, 86, 104
Non-maleficence, 84
Non-operative management (NOM), 8, 9
Non-prostate genitourinary cancers, 64
Non-small cell lung cancer (NSCLC), 4, 6, 8, 12, 21, 26, 30, 39, 63, 98, 145

No radiation therapy (NO-RT), **15**, 20
AI in patient selection for, 34–35
algorithm for determining, *78*
application of, 12, 81–82
appropriateness of, 6
balancing efficacy and safety, 41
barriers to international adoption of, 125–127
building network, 142–143
case for, 8–9
changing paradigm to, *4*
clinical case studies, 41
clinical trial evidence on, 38
clinical trials supporting, 92–93
collaborative movements, 14
complementary trials, 7–8
concept, 1–15
consensus statements, 12–13
cost-effectiveness of, 130–131
country-wise adoption, **129**
decision guidance tree for, *56*
decision-making process for, 12
emerging data, 7–8
ethical dilemmas in, 93
evolution of, *5*
expert opinions on, 121–122
feasibility of, 4
global perspectives on, 12
global trends, 14
goals, 14–15
identification of candidates, *76*
importance of, 41
influence of tumour biology on, 20–22
international collaboration, 144–145
international guidelines, 12–13
international perspectives on, 117
long-term outcomes of, 121
network, 142–143
in oncology, 154
outcomes, 7
overview, 2–3
patient groups ideal for, 81–82
policy shifts by 2030, 157
real-world data on, 94–95
risk–benefit analysis, 41
role in holistic cancer care, 152
role of AI/ML in decision-making of, 105
studies, 9–11
success in PMBCL, 115
support for, 7
surgical techniques in, 52–54
technological innovations, 41
vs. traditional RT, 120
treatment paradigms impact, 14
trial design, 7
Number needed to treat (NNT), 96
Nutritional support, 66, 72

O

Obesity, 82; *see also* Type 2 diabetes
Omission of radiation therapy, 112, 115, 119–120, 128–129
Oncologic surgery, 90
Oncologist, 141
Oncotype DX, 22, 33
Operational efficiencies, 130
OPRA trial, 8, 9
Optimized treatment planning, 137
Organ preservation, 50
Organ preservation in patients with rectal adenocarcinoma (OPRA), 3
Organ-sparing surgery, 53–54; *see also* Surgery
Osteosarcoma, 63
Overall survival (OS), 6, 50, 112, 139

P

Paediatric patients, 40
Pancreatic cancer, 8, 10, 28, 62, 66, 72, 83
Paradigms, changing, 3–6
Partial breast irradiation (PBI), 85
Pathological complete response (pCR), 8
Pathologist, 141
Patient-centric approaches, 100–101
cancer-specific strategies, 101
documentation/data collection, 101–102
evidence-based recommendations, 101
follow-up protocols, 101
holistic care, 100
individualized surveillance, 101
real-world compliance, 100
survival and quality of life, 101
telehealth options, 100
Patient-reported outcomes (PROs), 55, 68
Patients
autonomy, 84, 93
centred care, 67–68
centred data, 83
centred decision-making, 116
centred outcomes, 58
immunocompromised, 82, 86
management, 125
outcomes, 65–66, 95, 97, 131

preference, 52
risk assessing tools/techniques, 79–80
selection, 123
support, 137
Patient selection standards, 76–86
ethical considerations, 83–84
LUMINA trial, 84
multidisciplinary evaluation, 82–83
patient profiles, 81–82
risk stratification, 79–80
selection criteria, 76–77
PD-L1 expression, 20–22, 30, 32, 33–34
Pelvic radiation therapy, 50
Penetration depth, 132
Photodynamic therapy (PDT), 132
Policy changes, 155–156
Positron emission tomography (PET), 26
Postmastectomy, 29, 77
Postmastectomy radiation therapy (PMRT), 104
Postoperative care, 141
Postoperative radiation, 9
Precision medicine, 29, 80, 86, 99, 104, 113, 117, 118–119, 131, 155
Precision oncology, investment in, 131
PRECISION-RT trial, 14
Primary mediastinal B-cell lymphoma (PMBCL), 111–113, 115, 117, 118, 119, 121
PRIME II trial, 9, 11, 38, 41, 57
Proficient mismatch repair (pMMR), 31
Prognostic biomarkers, 30–32
Progression-free survival (PFS), 8, 112
PROSPECT trial, 50, 51, 55–56
Prostate cancer, 66, 130
decipher score in, 33
economic modelling in, 130
treatment controversies, 127
Prostate-specific membrane antigen (PSMA), 137
Proton beam radiotherapy (PBRT), 28, 73
Proton beam therapy, 120
Proton therapy, 63, 64–65, 67, 68
PULS-Pal trial, 92

Q

Quality-adjusted life years (QALYs), 6, 7
Quality assurance (QA), 124
Quality of life (QoL), 2, 6, 8, 12, 101, 155
benefits, 73
considerations, 34–35, 145
enhanced, 152
improving, 9
metrics, 11, 154
of patients, 52
post-treatment, 4
QUARTZ trial, 6–8

R

Radiation
decreasing reliance on, 3
exposure reduction, 95
induced toxicity, 2
related toxicities, 50
Radiation Oncology Collection (ROC), 9
Radiation therapy (RT)/radiotherapy, **15**
benefits of, 28
in close margin cases, 90–91
de-escalation of, 7
evolution of, 4, *5*
genetic resistance to, 52
long-term risks of, 28
long-term toxicity of, 52
need, 20–42
overview of, 1–2
risks associated with, 29
role, 1
targeted therapies as alternatives to, 62–63
Radioactive iodine (RAI), 120
Radiochemotherapy, 77
Radiofrequency ablation (RFA), 39, 63, 64, 68–69
Radiologist, 141
Radiotherapist, 141
Randomized controlled trials, 153
RAPIDO trial, 121
R-CHOP regimen, 117
Real-world compliance, 100
Real-world data (RWD), 94–95
data-driven decision-making, 95
enhanced patient outcomes, 95
reduction in radiation exposure, 95
Rectal cancer, 81, 121; *see also* Cancer
neoadjuvant chemotherapy for locally advanced, 55–56
pathway algorithm, 104
treatment approaches, 128
watch-and-wait strategy in, 56
Reduced morbidity, 152
Regulatory variability, 125
Reimbursement, 155–156
Resectable tumours, 52; *see also* Tumours
Resource allocation, 130

Risk
balancing, 94
vs. benefit, 28–29
Risk stratification, 79–80
breast cancer, 80
examples of, 80–81
in neoadjuvant therapy, 81
patient selection standards, 79–80
in rectal cancer, 81
Robotic-assisted surgery, 53; *see also* Surgery
Robust clinical evidence, 115
Roentgen, Wilhelm Conrad, 1
Roentgen-based dosimetry system, 1
Royal Marsden Hospital, case study, 117–119

S

Sammartino, P., 104
Second-line chemotherapy, 11; *see also* Chemotherapy
Selective targeting, 133
Sentinel lymph node biopsy (SLNB), 54
Sequelae, assessment of, 123
Shared decision-making, 94, 145; *see also* Decision-making
Short tandem repeats (STRs), 29
Single-nucleotide polymorphisms (SNPs), 29
Sjögren, T., 1
Small- and medium-sized enterprises (SMEs), 142
Small cell lung cancer (SCLC), 7
Smith, Jane, 121
Smith, J.J., 56
Soft tissue sarcoma (STS), 12
Specialty care networks, 140
Standard external beam radiation therapy (STND), 120
Standardization, 126
Standardized reporting, 138
Stenbeck, T., 1
Stereotactic body radiation therapy (SBRT), 28, 120
Stereotactic radiosurgery (SRS), 7
Stereotactic radiotherapy (SRT), 7
Strategic funding, 131
Structured algorithms, 89–90
Surgery, 90–91
as alternative to RT, 50
cytoreductive, 54
laparoscopic, 53
organ-sparing, 53–54
overview, 49
preferred over radiotherapy, 52
vs. radiation, **54**
robotic-assisted, 53
significance in tumour management, 49–58
trials, 51, **51**
Surgical advancements timeline, *49*
Surgical oncology, 50
Surgical resection, 50
Surgical *vs.* radiation, *55*
Systemic chemotherapy, 8; *see also* Chemotherapy
Systemic therapies, 62–63

T

Tang, Y., 80, 104
Targeted therapies, 62–63
TARGIT-A trial, 90, 91–92
Team-based approach, 136–138
coordination of care, 137–138
enhanced patient support, 137
improved diagnostic accuracy, 136
optimized treatment planning, 137
Technological advancements, 152
Technology limitations, 131
Technology transfer, 70, 71
Telehealth options, 100
Three-dimensional conformal radiotherapy (3DCRT), 28
Time-to-benefit (TTB), 96
Total mesorectal excision (TME), 8, 41, 50, 113, 114
Total neoadjuvant therapy (TNT), 3, 121, 128
Toxicity, 62
Training challenges, 126
Transanal total mesorectal excision (TaTME), 50
Transarterial chemoembolization (TACE), 65
Transcatheter aortic valve replacement (TAVR), 79
Transurethral resection of the bladder tumour (TURBT), 53–54
Treatment
cost-effective paradigm, 22
costs, 130
optimization, 35–36
paradigms impact, 14
planning and execution, 123–124
Trial design, 7, 92, 154
Trial master file (TMF), 102
Triple-negative breast cancer (TNBC), 2, 27
Tumour-associated macrophages (TAMs), 24
Tumour biology, 20–42
abscopal effect considerations, 40
adaptive radiotherapy, 35–36
in breast cancer, 40
cancer-associated fibroblasts (CAFs), 28
decision-making based on, *21*
dose painting, 35–36

factors influencing treatment decisions, 40–41
hypoxic tumour response, 26, *27*
immune cell interaction, 27
impact on treatment, 33–34
influence of, 20–22
multicriteria optimization, 36
optimization advances, 36
overview, 20
real-time adaptive techniques, 36–37
risk *vs.* benefit, 28–29
technical details, 36–37
technical innovations, 35–36
treatment optimization, 35–36
treatment response, 23–24
trials and outcomes, 38–39, **39**
tumour microenvironment (TME), 23–24
understanding, 23
Tumour microenvironment (TME), *23*, 23–24, *25*, 26
Tumours
age and, 38
behaviour, 29
board discussions, 91
board meetings, 138–139
central nervous system, 73
characteristics, 40–41, 114
characteristics analysis, 28
decision-making for treatment strategies, *31*
early-stage breast cancer, 37
evolution of, 25–26
genetic characteristics of, 24–25
HER2-negative, 2
heterogeneity, 25–26, 42, 100
implications for treatment, 38
induced metastasis risks, 40
localized, 52
molecular characteristics of, 24–25
resectable, 52, 53
surgery significance in, 49–58
types, 37–38
Type 2 diabetes, 82; *see also* Obesity

U

Ultrasound-guided superficial radiotherapy (US-SRT), 120
Urinary fistulae, 29
Urological complications, 29

V

Video-assisted thoracoscopic surgery (VATS), 50
Virtual tumour boards, 140
Vitzthum, L.K., 104

W

Watch-and-wait (W&W) strategy, 8, 56, 113, 119, 128
case study, 56, 113–115
challenges in implementing, 115–116
Whole-brain radiotherapy (WBRT), 6, 7
Whole breast irradiation (WBI), 85
Workflow adaptation, 124
Workforce challenges, 126
World Health Organization (WHO), 70, 78, 127

For Product Safety Concerns and Information please contact our
EU representative GPSR@taylorandfrancis.com Taylor & Francis
Verlag GmbH, Kaufingerstraße 24, 80331 München, Germany